D0486795

The New Book of
MASSAGE

CITY COLLEGE MANCHESTER

00029134

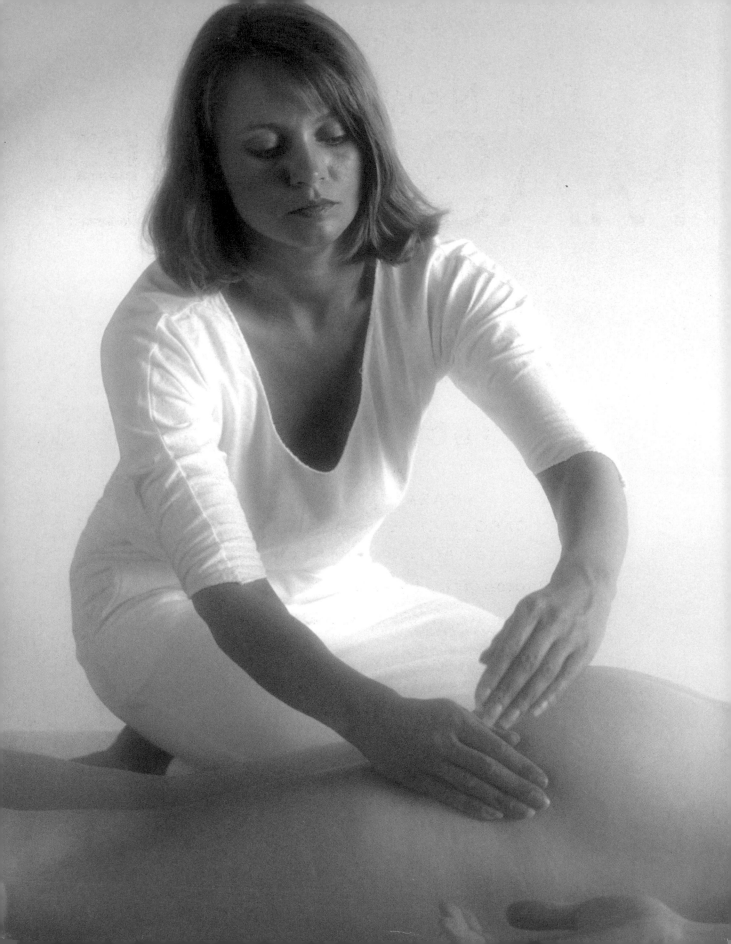

The New Book of
MASSAGE

Revised Edition of the Bestselling Step-by-Step Guide to Eastern and Western Techniques

LUCY LIDELL

with

SARA THOMAS

CAROLA BERESFORD-COOKE

and ANTHONY PORTER

Photography by FAUSTO DORELLI

Foreword by CLARE MAXWELL-HUDSON

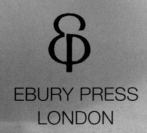

EBURY PRESS
LONDON

A GAIA ORIGINAL

Written by Lucy Lidell

with Sara Thomas *(massage)*
Carola Beresford-Cooke *(shiatsu)*
and Anthony Porter *(reflexology)*

Photography by Fausto Dorelli

Managing editor: Pip Morgan

Editorial and layout preparation: Aardvark Editorial

Design revisions: Patrick Nugent

Illustrations: Joe Robinson

Illustration revisions: Sheilagh Noble

Direction: Joss Pearson, Patrick Nugent

This revised edition of *The Book of Massage*
published in Great Britain in 2000
by Ebury Press, Random House,
20 Vauxhall Bridge Road, London SW1V 2SA
www.randomhouse.co.uk

Random House Australia (Pty) Limited,
20 Alfred Street, Milsons Point, Sydney,
New South Wales 2061, Australia

Random House New Zealand Limited,
18 Poland Road, Glenfield, Auckland 10, New Zealand

Random House (Pty) Limited,
Endulini, 5a Jubilee Road, Parktown 2193, South Africa

for Random House UK Limited Reg. No. 954009

Copyright © Gaia Books Limited 2000

All rights reserved. No part of this publication may be reproduced,
stored in a retrieval system, or transmitted in any form or by any means,
electronic, mechanical, photocopying, recording or otherwise, without
the prior written permission of the copyright owner.

A CIP catalogue record for this book is available from the British Library

ISBN 0–09–187843–8

Printed in Italy by Printer Trento

Note: If you have a medical condition, or are pregnant,
the exercises described in this book should not be
followed without first consulting your doctor. All guidelines
and warnings should be read carefully and the authors
and publishers cannot accept responsibility for injuries or
damage arising out of a failure to comply with the same.

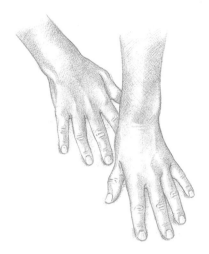

About this book...

Three different therapies are taught in *The New Book of Massage* – massage, shiatsu and reflexology. Whichever you decide to learn, please be sure to read Beginning (pp. 18–25), which contains practical advice that is fundamental to all three, and the Human Touch (pp. 152–65), which shows you how to apply the techniques to a range of ages and special needs.

Note: In the Massage section, receivers are shown naked, since the book is intended mainly for use with partners and close friends. In professional massage, you would always use towels to cover the body (see pp. 38–9).

Caution: Always consult a doctor if you are in doubt about a medical condition, and observe the cautions and contraindications given in the book.

Foreword

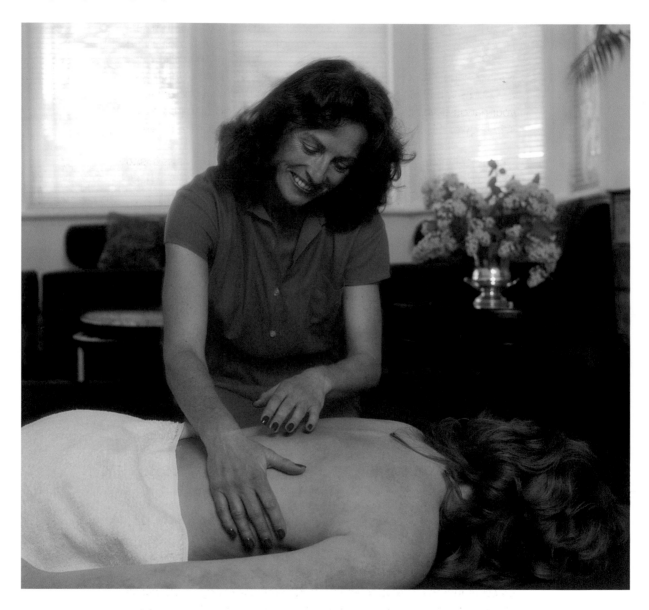

Massage is perhaps the oldest and simplest of all medical treatments. In traditional cultures, especially in the East, it is accepted as natural that people of all ages can benefit from regular massage. But here in the West, although its value has always been recognized in the world of sport, its use has only quite recently spread to other fields.

All too often, we tend to be afraid to touch one another. Yet increasingly, research is proving the extraordinary effectiveness of touch – and touch is the core of massage. In a recent survey, the simple act of massage was shown to have improved patients' morale, and hastened their rate of recovery. I myself have found this to be true in my own hospital work.

For massage, as one discovers during its practice, is not only physical. It contains much of psychology. Understanding of the person under your hands develops through empathy. As every good therapist in the field knows, this is rooted in the inward resolution: "I am here to help."

One unique advantage is that massage is as pleasant to give as it is to receive. It has been scientifically established that stroking a household pet has a relaxing effect and lowers one's blood pressure. Stroking people does the same.

Massage can be stimulating or soothing, depending on the speed and depth of your strokes. This is why it can make a person feel alert and ready to run in a marathon – or, conversely, relaxed and sleepy. It can relieve tension, soothe away headaches, relax taut and aching muscles and banish insomnia. Above all, it can provide a context for recovery by inducing a sense of well-being. Many of my clients are sure that the pleasure it gives is therapeutic in itself.

Yet with all these benefits, massage is easy to learn. It is a skill that everyone can acquire because it is, fundamentally, an extension of something we all do instinctively. We stroke our foreheads when tired or headachey, we pat our children on the head or face to reassure them, we hold a friend's hand in comfort and we rub a painful area as inevitably as we stroke our pets. The aim of this book is to help you develop this natural capacity.

Massage may be defined as any systematic form of touch which has been found to give comfort or to promote good health. In this book three different techniques are described: massage as such, where the strokes are generally large and flowing; shiatsu, an Oriental method of pressure therapy, related to acupuncture; and reflexology, which affects all parts of the body by working on reflexes in the feet. *The New Book of Massage* is thus an excellent introduction to the subject. With its help anyone can start to develop the therapeutic powers in their hands.

Remember, life may take it out of you, but massage can put it back.

Contents

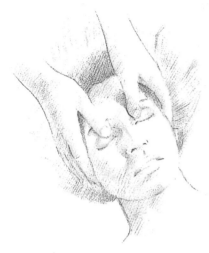

10 Introduction

18 Beginning

20 Creating a Relaxed Environment

22 Giving and Receiving

24 Centring

26 Massage

28 Oiling

30 Basic Strokes

36 Basic Massage Sequence

38 Towels and Padding

40 The Back

46 Back of Legs

52 Shoulders, Neck and Scalp

58 The Face

63 Arms and Hands

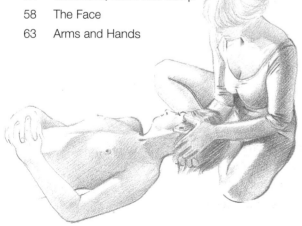

68 Front of Torso

72 Front of Legs

76 Connecting

78 Massage Checklist

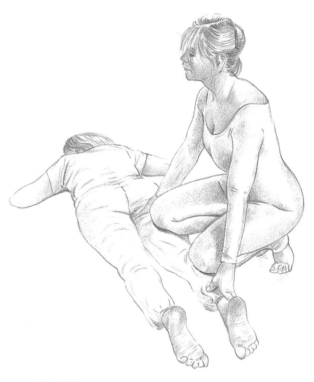

80 Shiatsu

82 *Ki*

86 The Oriental Way of Health

88 Tools and Techniques

90 Basic Shiatsu Sequence

92 The Back

96 The Hips

100 Back and Outside of Legs

106 Back of Shoulders

110 Front of Shoulders and Neck

114 Head and Face

118 Arms and Hands

122 The *Hara*

126 Front and Inside of Legs

130 Shiatsu Checklist

131 Pressure Points for Massage

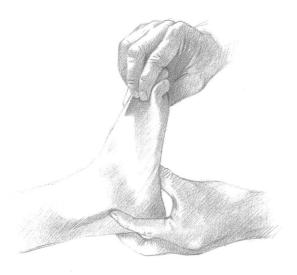

132 Reflexology

134 Theory and Principles
136 Foot Reflexes Chart
138 Basic Techniques
142 Foot Treatment Sequence
148 Hand Reflexes Chart
150 Hand Treatment Sequence

152 The Human Touch

154 Maternity
156 Babies
160 Later Life
162 Massage and Exercise
164 Self-massage

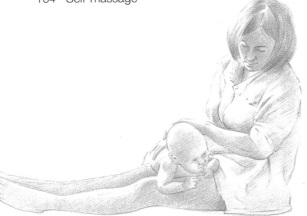

166 Body Reading

168 Splits and Asymmetries
170 Feet and Legs
172 The Pelvis/The Belly
174 The Chest/Shoulders and Arms

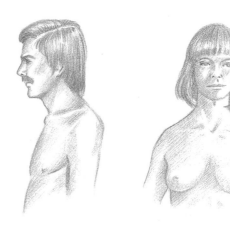

176 Neck, Head, and Face
178 The Body Speaks

180 Anatomy

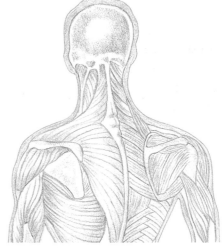

190 Recommended Reading
190 Useful Addresses
191 Index
192 Acknowledgments

Introduction

Everyone needs to relax, to escape the tyranny of time. Listening to music, watching the movements of clouds, combing the beach for pebbles or shells – these are all ways we use to still the mind, to regain a sense of our own wholeness in the innocence of the moment. As children we climb trees and run around barefoot. We are at home with ourselves and in touch with our basic nature. But as we grow older we spend more and more time living purely in our heads.

Now is the time to redress the balance and get back into your body by rediscovering the gentle art of touch. It is a common language, one that we can use to heal or reassure, to relieve pain or soothe away tension – above all, to convey the fact that we care. Like a clearing in the forest, it gives us a breathing space in which to relax and reorientate ourselves.

Massage can provide us with a means to counteract the relentless surge of work and domestic pressures. For all too many of us, stiffness and pain are a way of life to which we have become habituated, and it is often not until we give or receive massage that we realize that our muscles are tight, or come to see how much of our energy is consumed by tension. Massage can be a voyage of self-discovery, revealing how it feels to be more relaxed and in tune with ourselves, to experience the pleasure of a body that can breathe, stand and move freely.

Massage, Past and Present

For thousands of years some form of massage or laying on of hands has been used to heal and soothe the sick. To the ancient Greek and Roman physicians, massage was one of the principal means of relieving pain. In the early fifth century BC, Hippocrates – the "father of medicine" – wrote: "The physician must be experienced in many things, but assuredly in rubbing... For rubbing can bind a joint that is too loose, and loosen a joint that is too rigid."

Pliny, the renowned Roman naturalist, was regularly rubbed to relieve his asthma, and Julius Caesar, who suffered from epilepsy, was daily pinched all over, to ease his neuralgia and headaches. After the fall of Rome in the fifth century AD, little progress was made in Europe in the sphere of medicine and it was left to the Arabs to study and develop the teachings of the classical world. Avicenna, the eleventh-century Arab philosopher and physician, noted in his *Canon* that the object of massage was "to disperse the effete matters found in the muscles and not expelled by exercise".

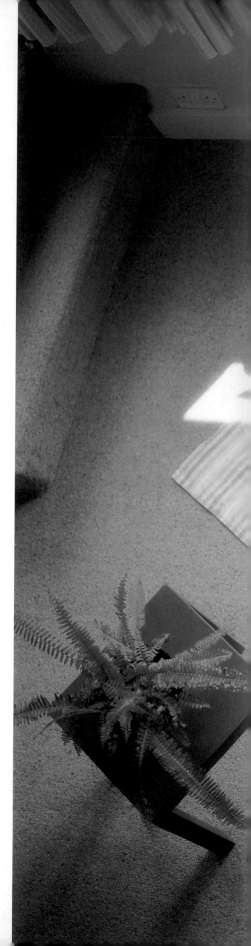

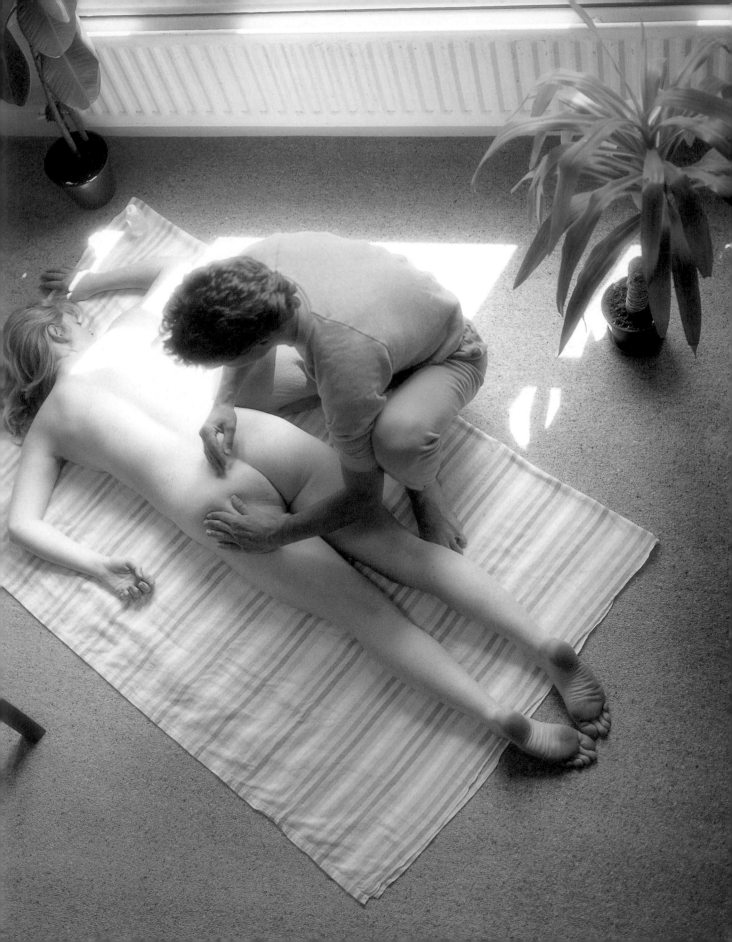

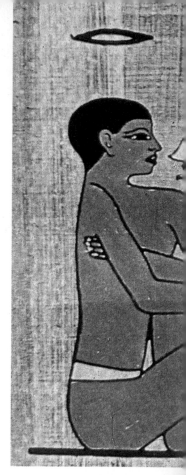

During the Middle Ages, in Europe, little was heard of massage, due to the contempt for the pleasures of the flesh. But it was revived in the sixteenth century, mainly through the work of a French doctor, Ambroise Paré. Then, at the beginning of the nineteenth century, a Swede by the name of Per Henrik Ling developed what is now known as Swedish massage, synthesizing his system from his knowledge of gymnastics and physiology and from Chinese, Egyptian, Greek and Roman techniques. In 1813 the first college offering massage as part of the curriculum was established in Stockholm and from then on institutes and spas that included massage sprang up all over the continent. Today, the therapeutic value of massage has once more been recognized, and it continues to flourish and develop throughout the Western world, both among lay practitioners and professionals.

In the East, massage techniques have always been more valued for their healing applications than in the West and their use has continued in an unbroken line since earliest times. Perhaps the difference that has until very recently existed between Eastern and Western attitudes to massage stems from the scientific revolution which took place in the West some 250 years ago. As a result of this new science, older concepts which linked the body to the mind and spirit were discounted as unscientific and, in the course of time, the human body came to be regarded as a kind of sophisticated machine, which could be serviced and maintained only by highly trained and specialized people – in other words, doctors.

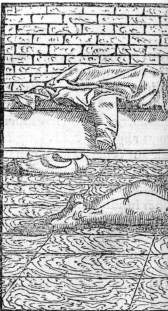

In the East, however, no such "scientific" attitude took root until very recently, and the poor country people continued to combine the instinctive desire to "rub it better" with skills refined and elaborated by long tradition and lent authority by a "barefoot doctor" knowledge of Oriental medical theory and bonesetting or manipulative techniques. Shiatsu originated from this traditional type of massage, as practised in Japan, and as it gained recognition it became enriched by further influences from classical acupuncture theory, and from the Western sciences of osteopathy and chiropractic newly arrived in Japan. The beginnings of reflexology are unknown – it may well have sprung from the ancient art of Oriental pressure point therapy. But, whatever its precise origins, it seems certain that it was in use in ancient Egypt, as evidenced by the wall paintings from a physician's tomb, shown above right.

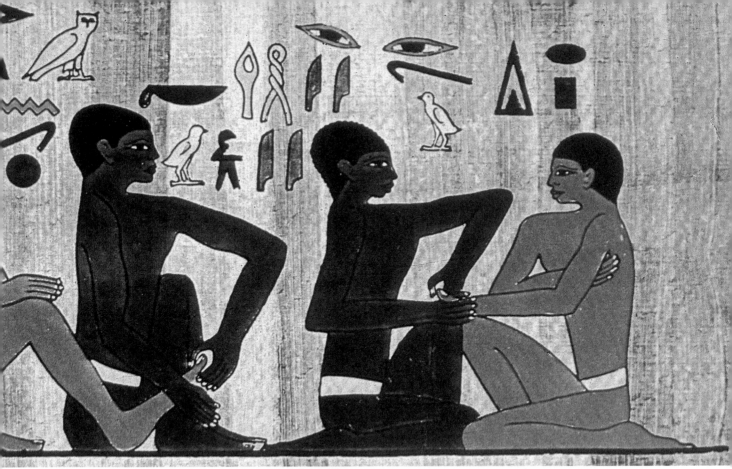

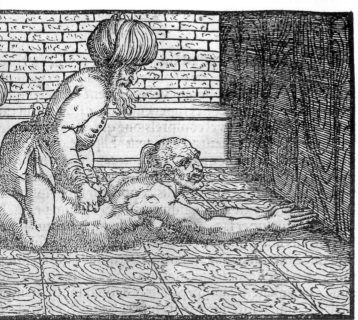

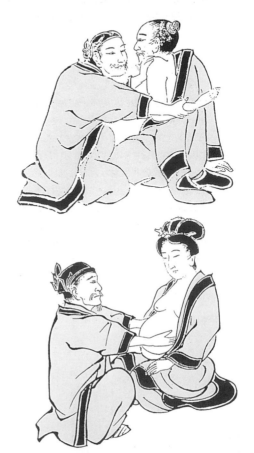

Historical evidence of reflexology, massage and shiatsu: top, wall painting from a physician's tomb in Saqqara, Egypt, dating from 2330 BC; above, illustration from the Canon of Avicenna (980–1037 AD); right, adaptations of woodcuts taken from an early nineteenth-century Japanese text.

The Language of Touch

Touch means contact – the relationship with what lies outside our own periphery, the ground beneath our feet. And for humans, as for other animals, touch is of vital importance. It gives reassurance, warmth, pleasure, comfort and renewed vitality. It tells us we are not alone.

Of all the senses, touch is the first to develop. As babies, it is primarily through our tactile experience that we explore and make sense of the world, and the loving touch of our parents is essential to our growth. As long as our need to touch and be touched is satisfied, we grow healthy, but where it is inhibited, so our development may be impaired. The cuddles and strokes we receive in infancy help us to build a healthy image of ourselves, nurturing the feeling that, because we are touched, we are accepted and loved. Over 35 years ago, the American psychologist S.M. Jourard showed that our perception of how much we are touched by other people seems to be clearly related to our self-esteem, to how much we value ourselves.

Experiments with infant primates have proved how essential physical contact with a warm, caring mother is, and, conversely, how physically and emotionally stunting touch deprivation can be, for our entire sense of reality is based on the sense of touch. In our society, to be deprived of contact with our fellow men is a punishment – the worst of all being solitary confinement. When we are prevented from touching or being touched we feel painfully alone and anxious. In a recent American medical study, patients denied skin contact reported feeling acutely isolated, cut off from the warmth of human touch.

Touch is a language we all use instinctively to show our feelings, to demonstrate to others that they are loved, wanted or appreciated. "Let's rub it better" is our natural response to a child's bumps and bruises; hands move swiftly to rest on fevered brows or to soothe sore tummies and headaches. Emotional pain too evokes an immediate response. Holding, comforting, stroking, we convey sympathy, understanding, reassurance. Alone and in pain we cradle and hug ourselves, rest tired heads in hands, unconsciously massage our aching limbs. But aside from perhaps embracing one another purely in friendship, to convey our happiness and joy, have we not strayed far from our instincts by reserving the language of touch for cries of pain and sorrow or for the context of sex – by being afraid to touch merely to express affection, to relax or to heal?

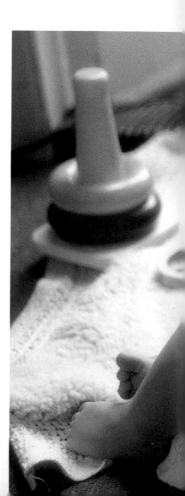

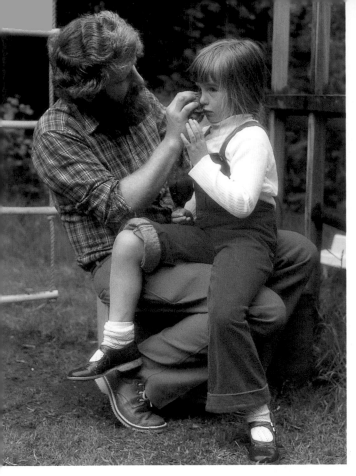
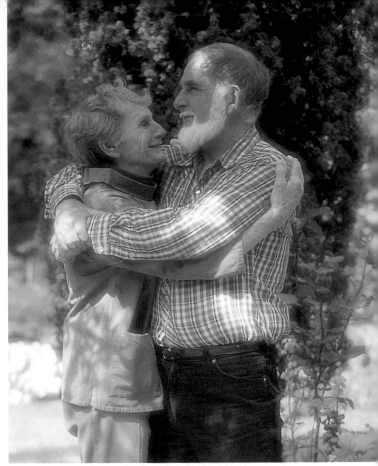
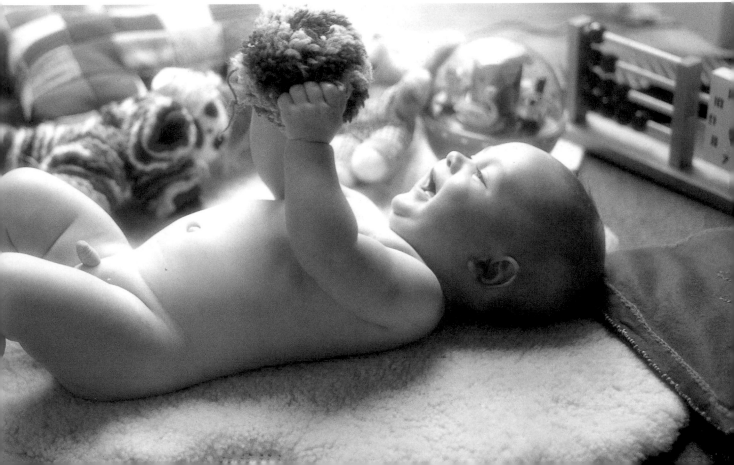

Massage, Shiatsu, and Reflexology

In this book we will show how touch techniques can be used not only to relax and increase the well-being of family and friends, but also to enhance your understanding of yourself and others. The three touch therapies presented – massage, shiatsu, and reflexology – differ greatly in effect and mode of application. All three, however, work with the body's regenerative capacity, promoting each individual's own self-healing ability. We suggest that you start by learning the therapy to which you feel temperamentally most drawn – of these, massage is perhaps the easiest to learn, for its movements elaborate on strokes that we all do naturally. Shiatsu and reflexology need a more precise approach than massage.

Massage involves systematically stroking, kneading and pressing the soft tissues of the entire body in order to induce a state of total relaxation. The receiver is naked or partially clothed, and oil is used to lubricate the skin. Once you have learned the basic sequence of strokes, you can begin to work more with your intuition, adapting the techniques according to the receiver's needs. In massage, your hands flow continuously over broad areas of the body, whereas in shiatsu and reflexology you work most of the time with pressure on small areas or points.

Shiatsu is a Japanese system of physical therapy, given with the fingers, thumbs, elbows, knees, or feet. It differs from massage in the principle on which it is based. Whereas massage works mainly on the muscles, ligaments and tendons, and particularly affects the body's fluid balance of blood and lymph, shiatsu involves concentrating on pressure points or tsubos, in order to affect the balance of vital energy or ki in the meridians. Since both therapies involve working over the whole body, shiatsu will also incidentally affect the muscular, circulatory and lymphatic systems, just as massage will affect the pressure points and meridians, even if not by design. Shiatsu is usually received with the clothes on – partly for reasons of modesty, since the treatment involves moving the receiver's limbs into some fairly exposed positions. It is particularly effective as preventive medicine and as a pick-me-up for people who are run down or convalescing after an illness.

In reflexology, you use special thumb and finger techniques to work on small areas, or reflexes, on the feet. These reflex areas are connected to different parts of the body, so that in working over all the reflexes on the feet you are in fact affecting the entire body. The main benefit of reflexology is relaxation, but it also improves the blood supply and the functioning of nerve impulses.

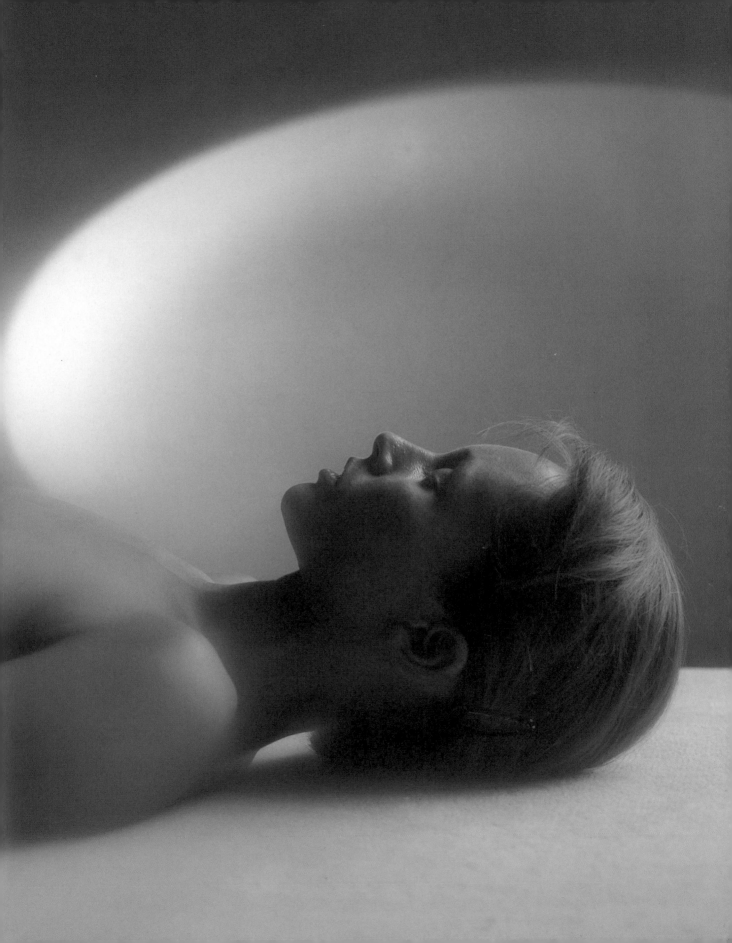

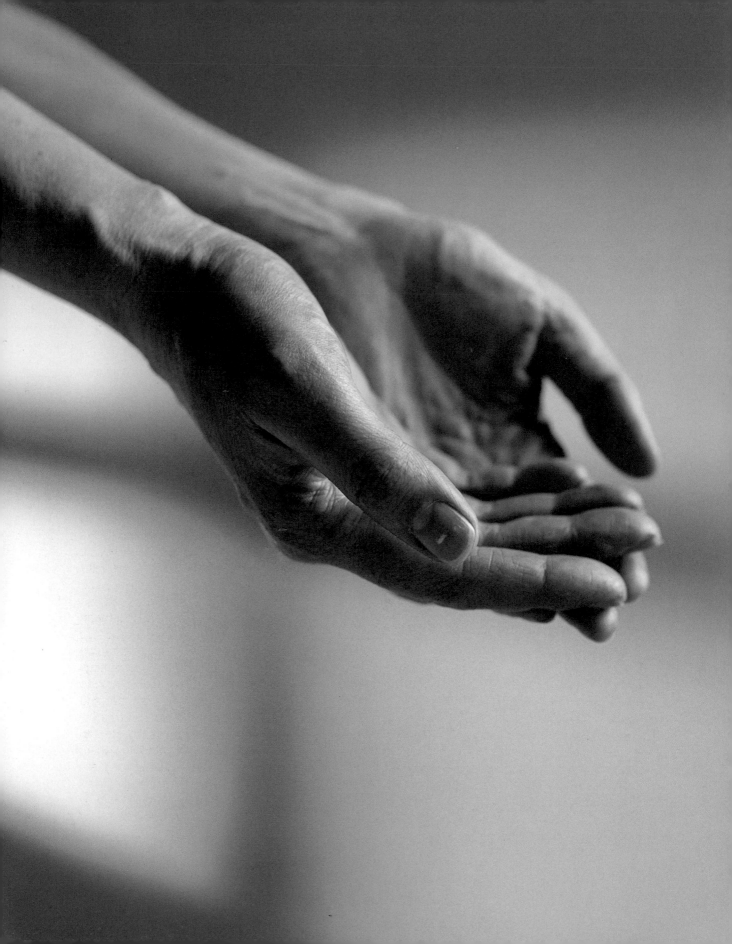

Beginning

Care and sensitivity, a little time and energy, and a good pair of hands – this is all that's needed to begin practising massage. But no matter which of the touch therapies you choose to learn, there are certain important guidelines for treatment that apply to all three.

First, it is worth taking the trouble to set the scene in advance, so that you are well prepared for the session before you begin – with the room already warm and snug, pillows, cushions, blankets and towels available, and any oil or powder you may need at hand. You will break the flow of the treatment if you have to stop to go in search of another heater, or more oil. And you will defeat the whole object of the exercise if your partner cannot relax because he or she is chilly or uncomfortable. Think about what you will need for your own comfort, too. To give good massage or shiatsu, it is essential to wear clothes that allow you to move freely. And each time you change positions within a treatment session, you must make sure that you feel relaxed, not strained, before carrying on with the treatment. Never make do with a slightly awkward position, thinking that the discomfort will disappear. It won't, and your tension will be transmitted to your partner.

As the giver, your comfort is closely linked to your posture and breathing. Whether you are sitting, kneeling or standing, your body should feel balanced and relaxed. To allow the healing energy to flow freely, keep your back straight rather than stooping or bending, and move from your belly and pelvis, using your whole body to apply pressure, not just your hands or shoulders. If you can breathe fully and let your body "dance" as you move, you will avoid getting tense or tired and will end a treatment with as much energy as when you started.

Central to the success of any touch therapy is your state of mind and attitude to your partner. You should regard each session as a new experience and bring to each one a feeling of genuine caring, consideration and respect. Before giving a treatment, talk to the receiver about what you are going to do and find out if there are any special problems. Encourage your partner to interrupt you during the session if he or she is uncomfortable or if your pressure is too light or too strong. But in general discourage chatting. You will only lose your concentration and may well sacrifice the preciousness of quiet focused touch to the overused language of every day. Never attempt to give a treatment if you are upset, angry, or unwell – for not only will your energy be depleted, but your mood will affect your partner.

It will help you to maintain the right attitude if you can stay "centred" and give your partner your full attention. Many of us spend much of our lives thinking of the past or idly worrying about the future, and miss what is going on in the present moment. For all touch therapies it is essential that you keep your attention on the "here and now", for the healing energy transmitted through your hands will be weakened or deflected by an absent mind. When you are centred, you are guided by your intuition and will more readily sense where the sources of tension or energy imbalance lie in your partner. You will be able to find the right touch for each part of the body, and to differentiate between a "good hurt" and excessive pressure. But if your thoughts do start to drift while you are working, simply bring them gently back and quieten your mind by concentrating on your breathing. Working with your eyes closed for brief periods may help you to stay in touch with what you are doing and keep your attention in your hands.

Creating a Relaxed Environment

Relaxation is central to any form of massage, and the more you can do to provide a calm, comfortable setting, the more effective your treatment will be. Whatever your home is like, it only takes a little care and preparation to transform part of it into a peaceful massage area. Probably the two most essential requirements are heat and quiet. The room you choose should be draught-free and very warm – particularly for an oil massage, when the receiver will be naked or partially clothed. For massage you will need a couple of large towels, to use as covering both during the session and at the end (see pp. 38–9). For shiatsu and reflexology, you should have a rug available, to cover your partner at the end. Make sure you have some pillows or small cushions at hand as well, to use as padding for your partner or yourself. Choose a time for giving massage when you and your partner can be quiet and undisturbed, so that your concentration remains unbroken. Some people like to play relaxing music in the background, others may find music of any kind intrusive. The lighting in the room should be soft and subdued, as bright lights prevent the eyes relaxing completely. The gentle glow of candlelight is ideal. As a final touch, you can use flowers or incense to add fragrance to the atmosphere.

Working Surfaces

Of the three touch techniques taught in this book, shiatsu is always given on the floor, holistic massage on the floor or on a massage table, and reflexology is given with the receiver sitting or lying back in a chair (see p. 138). For shiatsu, you need more space than for massage – at least 2.5 × 2 m (8.2 × 6.5 feet). If your floor is well carpeted, you need only spread out a folded blanket or duvet for the receiver, covered by a sheet or towel if you are giving an oil massage. But if the floor is hard, you will need extra padding. A futon or a large 2.5- to 5-cm-thick (1–2-inch) foam mattress is best, but if you don't have one, use additional layers of blankets or duvets. Make sure that the padding extends well beyond the receiver's body, to save your own knees as you move around. If you intend to do a lot of massage, it is worth investing in a massage table. Working on a table is less tiring, as you can easily reach all parts of the body without bending and can move around, without accidentally jogging your partner and interrupting the flow. Don't use a bed or spring mattress – any pressure you apply will be absorbed by the mattress.

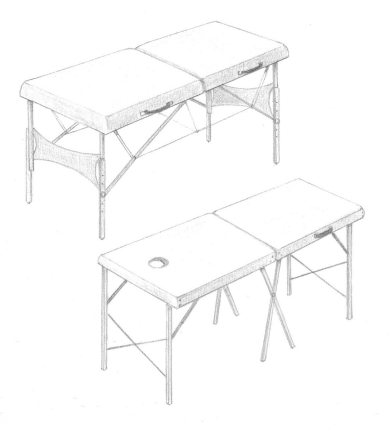

Massage Tables

There are many types of treatment couch available that are ideal for massage. Most are lightweight, folding and portable, often made of aluminium. Some are made with tension cables, providing excellent stability, and many have adjustable legs. To find the right height, you need to be able to brush the table top with the knuckles of a loosely swinging arm. All couches come with padded tops and many have built-in face holes, which allow receivers to lie face down without turning their heads. You can buy ready-made fitted couch covers or use a sheet or large towel to cover your table.

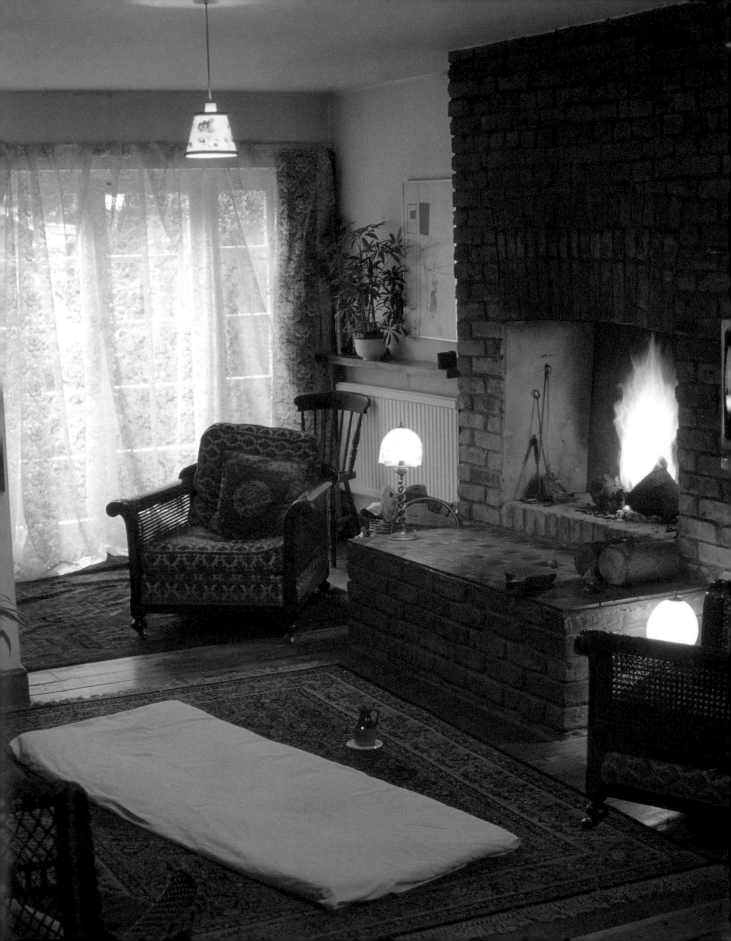

Giving and Receiving

Massage is a two-way flow of touch and response, a mutual exchange of energy. The hands, which both give and receive, and the skin – these are the instruments of communication. Through your hands you perceive and discover the uniqueness of the person you are touching; through their skin they receive the gift of your touch, the caring contact and movement. In a sense the terms "giver" and "receiver" are deceptive, since any form of touch therapy is a matter of sharing. For the healing power of touch to come through, both partners need to understand their roles in the exchange, both need to give and to be receptive – the receiver by giving his or her trust, by surrendering to the giver; the giver by being open and sensitive to the receiver's needs. At its highest level, massage can be a form of meditation, with both participants present in the moment, both focused on the point of contact between them. Practising the exercise below will allow you to experience touch given with focused awareness rather than mechanically.

Developing Sensitivity *(below)*
Sit down on the floor with your legs outstretched in front of you. Begin by centring your mind, then let your hands float gently down to make contact with one thigh. Now use your hands to stroke in broad sweeps and circles, focusing your awareness first in the heels of your hands (1), then in the palms (2), then in your thumbs (3), and finally in your fingers (4).

Focusing Your Awareness

To give good massage, body and mind need to be synchronized. The exercise (right) enables you to develop your sensitivity while giving and receiving touch simultaneously. It involves centring your awareness in different parts of your hands while you stroke down your leg. Each time you start by focusing your awareness in a part of your hands then briefly apply pressure with that part as you glide slowly down the leg. You need to keep your whole hand in touch with your skin, but let your full awareness remain in the chosen part. After a few minutes, you pause then repeat the process, transferring your awareness to a different part, as described above right.

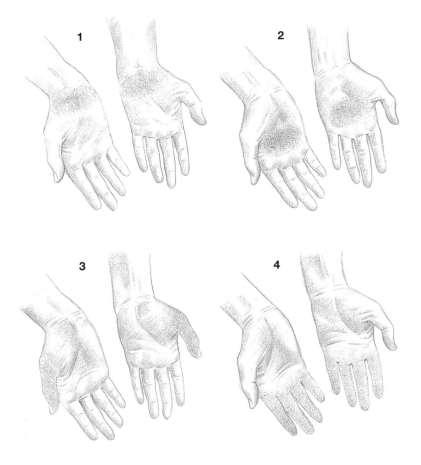

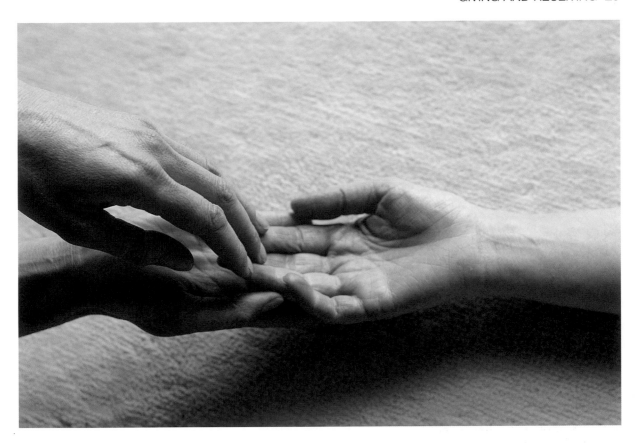

The Giver

It is important to be able to move freely when giving massage, so your clothes need to be comfortable, not restrictive. Before you begin a treatment, wash your hands and check that your fingernails are short. Take off your watch and any rings. Ask your partner to remove the necessary jewellery and clothes. If you are giving an oil massage to a partner or close friend, the receiver may choose to be naked, but you should always respect people's wishes if they feel happier partially clothed. Make the receiver comfortable, with padding under the ankles, upper chest, abdomen or knees, if required. And be sure to find a comfortable position before you begin centring yourself (see p. 25). During the treatment, try to keep your body relaxed and your mind focused on what you are doing. Always wash your hands at the end of the session.

The Receiver

To benefit fully from a massage, you need to play an active role in the healing process by paying attention to your partner's touch and keeping your mind free from wandering. As soon as you sit or lie down, let yourself melt down into the surface. Close your eyes and become aware of your breathing and the parts of your body that move as you inhale or exhale. Try to let go of any worries or problems that are on your mind. As you feel the giver's hands, be receptive and simply focus on the sensation engendered by his or her touch. Allow your limbs to be lifted and moved by the giver, surrendering rather than trying to help. Let the giver know if the pressure of touch is too deep, if anything feels uncomfortable – or if you are particularly enjoying a certain stroke or movement. But otherwise refrain from talking.

Centring

Centring is a way of focusing, of gathering your energy into a point so that you can channel it more easily into any activity you choose. It is a state of balance, quietness, strength and presence in the moment. More specifically, centring means focusing on the *hara*, the centre of energy in the abdomen, as shown opposite. For any form of massage, as for the martial arts, being centred in the *hara* is of primary importance as it enables you to be flexible yet resilient, to work with your intuition rather than your mind. When your energy is channelled from there, you need less muscle power and can give even a series of massage treatments without becoming tired or drained. Being centred is essentially linked to having the correct posture – with spine erect and neck and shoulders relaxed – and remaining "grounded" (see p. 170), or aware of your contact with the ground, through flexible legs and feet.

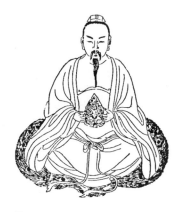

Breathing into the *Hara*
In Taoist yoga, one of the early stages of practice is a visualization and breathing meditation. The meditator concentrates on creating the eternal being in his hara *centre.*

The *Hara*

Hara is the Japanese word for belly or abdomen, known in Chinese as *tan t'ien* and in Arabic as *kath*. It refers to the source of vital energy and strength in the lower abdomen, more precisely to a point a few centimetres below the navel called the "Tan-Den" (see p. 122). The *hara* is the second of the "chakras", the seven energy centres, located mainly along the spine (see p. 189). Commonly regarded as the "earth" centre, it allows the energy from the earth to be gathered up into the pelvis, then relayed out via the arms and hands. It is our centre of gravity, power, equilibrium and stability, the nucleus of our physical and psychic powers. When practising any form of massage – or any of the martial arts – if you work "from the *hara*", your energy comes from your centre of gravity and you can operate without effort or strain (see p. 88).

The *Hara* in the Martial Arts
Someone who is centred in the hara, *like the karate master right, is powerful and immovable, like a tree whose roots go deep down into the earth. And with a strong centre, the energy can flow freely out through the arms and hands.*

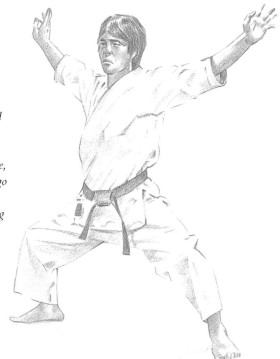

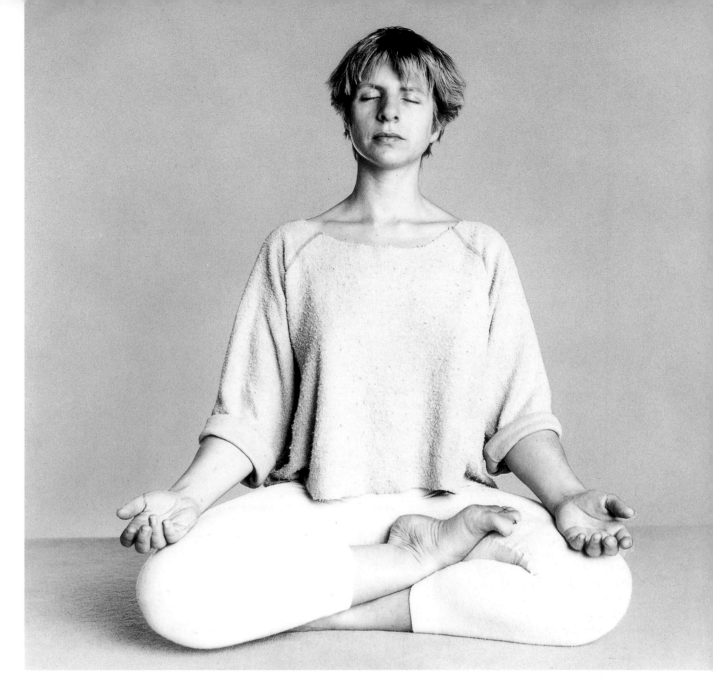

A Centring Meditation

Before giving any form of touch therapy – massage, shiatsu or reflexology – you should spend a few minutes centring yourself and connecting the energy between your *hara* and hands. Sit cross-legged or kneel down on the floor, putting a cushion under your buttocks, if necessary, to ease any strain on your legs. If you are still uncomfortable, sit on a straight-backed chair with both feet flat on the floor. Now close your eyes and direct your attention inward. Feel the strong foundation of your buttocks, legs and feet as they make contact with the cushion, chair or floor. From this firm base, allow your spine to float gently upward, without strain. Let go of any tension in your shoulders, neck and face. Now begin to focus on your breath, allowing it to find its own rhythm. Imagine that as you inhale, your breath fills your lower abdomen or *hara*. After a few breaths, begin also to visualize that, as you exhale, your breath flows up your torso from the *hara*, through your shoulders, down your arms, and out of your hands. If you wish, visualize the breath as a stream of energy or light flowing up the body and out of your fingers.

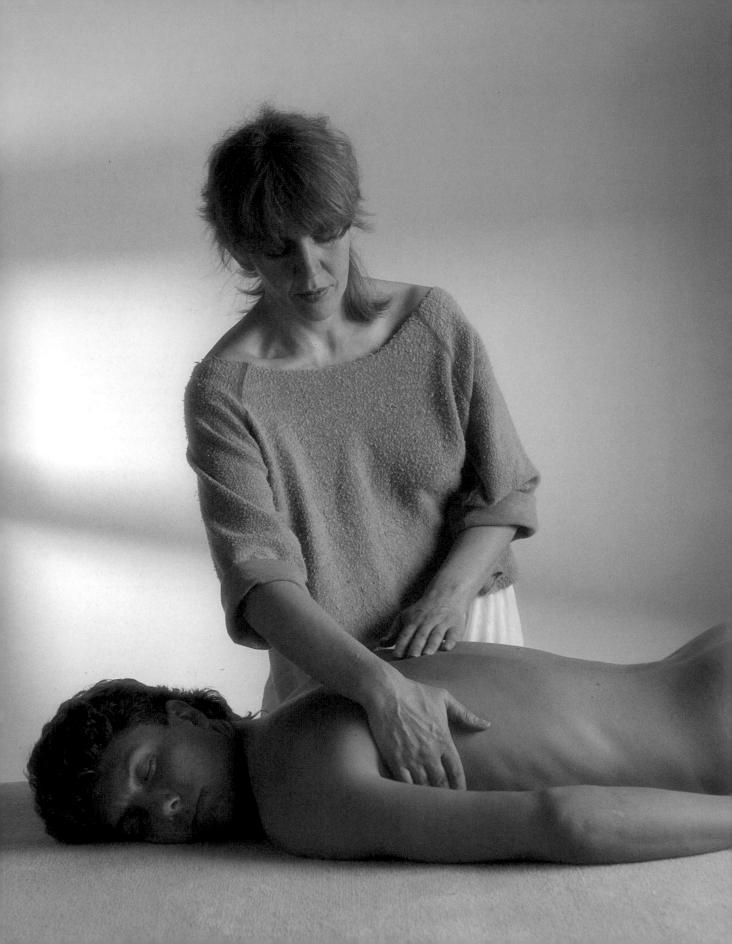

Massage

Massage is the sharing of touch – hands on body, on head, hands or feet. And yet massage goes farther than skin deep, deeper even than muscles and bones – a good, caring massage penetrates right to the depth of your being.

The kind of massage we are teaching here is often called holistic, or intuitive, massage, to distinguish it from sports and Swedish massage. Holistic massage treats the individual as a whole, rather than just concentrating on physical conditions, and its movements are generally slower and more meditative. In holistic massage, the attitude of both giver and receiver, and the communication between them, are of paramount importance to the effect of the treatment. The receiver's role is to be relaxed but alert, concentrating on the giver's touch, while the giver should try to remain centred and bring an attitude of genuine caring to the massage.

The basic massage we present in this chapter is divided into strokes and parts of the body in order to help you to learn, but it is not meant to be adhered to rigidly. To the receiver it should feel like one continuous sequence in which the strokes flow rhythmically from one to the other. Remember that any tension or awkwardness in your posture will be felt by your partner. If you practise letting your whole body move from the hips, rather than using just your arms and hands, you will soon find that your hands relax and the strokes begin to come naturally to you. With experience you will begin to improvise new strokes and develop your own language of touch as the body beneath your hands suggests possible movements.

When giving a massage, ask for feedback on what feels good, but avoid too much verbal communication, as talking will take your concentration away from your hands. The slower and more rhythmical your strokes are, the more relaxed and safe your partner will feel. Try to arrange to have a massage yourself while you are learning, so that you can experience different speeds and pressures of stroke for yourself.

A good massage affects you on all levels of your being. Physically, its benefits include relaxing and toning your muscles; assisting the venous flow of blood; soothing the nervous system; encouraging the lymphatic flow; and stretching the connective tissue of joints. Holistic massage also affects the energy centres or chakras of the "subtle body" (see p. 189). On a mental level, massage not only relieves stress and anxiety, it also helps you to become more conscious of your body as a whole, of the parts that you are in touch with and of those that feel "cut off". Once you are aware of where your energy blocks lie, you can begin to try and integrate your body and, in developing a more positive self-image, take responsibility for your own happiness and health.

A caring massage creates feelings of well-being, trust and joy. It can also release a great deal of energy hitherto wasted in tension and, by transforming chronic habits of acting and reacting, effect profound changes on both posture and facial expression (see Body Reading, pp. 166–79). The emotional aspect of massage is extremely important.

On a spiritual level, the benefits of massage are hard to describe, for we are talking of something that is intrinsically indefinable – the essence, the "life force", the whole that is more than the sum of its parts. But it is not uncommon during a holistic massage for both giver and receiver to attain a state of heightened awareness, of "presence in the moment", that is akin to the experience of meditation.

Oiling

As you come to work on each new part of the body, you begin by oiling it. This allows you to slide your hands smoothly and evenly over the contours without any risk of friction or jerkiness. It also nourishes the skin. Many people initially overestimate how much oil is needed – in fact, only a thin film is sufficient to lubricate the skin; if your partner's body is swimming in oil, you will be unable to make proper contact. For most parts of the body, a single application of oil is all that is necessary. But for larger expanses, like the back, or hairy areas, such as the front of the legs, you may need to apply extra oil. Since most oils are quickly absorbed by the skin, each part of the body is oiled separately, rather than all at once, with the oil rubbed into the skin by long gliding strokes.

Oils and Containers

There is no need to buy ready-made massage oils, which tend to be expensive. You can equally well use a vegetable oil, such as grapeseed, sunflower or safflower. Almond oil is very pleasant but costly; olive oil tends to be a little viscous. You can also use mineral oils, such as baby oil, although these are less easily absorbed. If you do use a plain oil, you may like to scent it with an essential oil, using five drops to an eggcupful of base oil. In aromatherapy, essential oils containing plant hormones are rubbed into the skin for specific therapeutic purposes. For those untrained in aromatherapy, it is best to stick to "safe" relaxing oils, such as lavender, chamomile or sandalwood, as some essential oils are contraindicated in certain conditions. Keep your oil in a corked bottle or a flip-top plastic bottle. The latter is more convenient as it is less likely to spill during a session. If you have nothing else, a bowl or saucer will do, but you must be careful not to knock it over, especially when working on the floor.

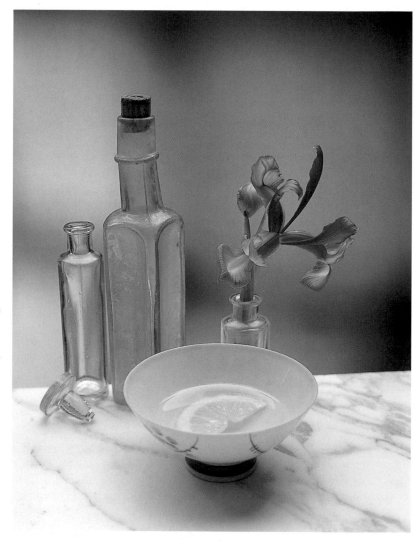

Preparations

It is at the very beginning of a massage that you set the mood for the whole session, so it pays to be well prepared. If possible, warm the oil beforehand – by standing the container in hot water or in front of a heater. And try to keep the oil in a safe place where you are unlikely to knock it over. Before applying the oil you should centre yourself (see p. 25), then let your hands rest briefly on your partner's head or body for the first gentle contact. Having established contact, pour about half a teaspoon of oil into one palm. You need to keep your hands well away from your partner's body while doing this, so that no stray drops accidentally fall on him or her.

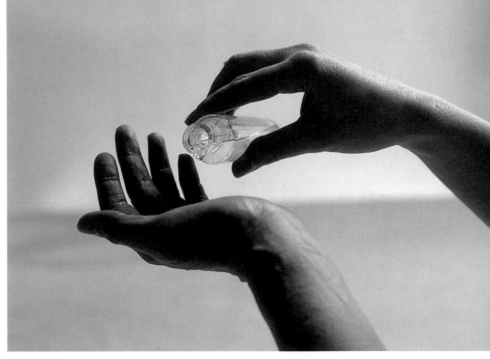

Applying Oil (*above*)
Holding your hands away from your partner's body, pour a little oil into one palm. Rub your palms together *to spread the oil, then bring them gently down and begin to apply the oil, using the long stroke (see p. 30).*

Making and Breaking Contact

The sensitivity with which you make and break contact with your partner is of prime importance. After oiling your hands, let them float slowly down toward the part of the body you are about to massage, as if suspended from parachutes. Just as you may feel the heat or energy that surrounds the body before you actually touch the skin, so your partner may sense the presence of your hands above his or her body. Make sure your hands are relaxed when they touch the body and, when you need to collect more oil or move to a new part of the body, let the break of contact be smooth and gentle too. Some schools of massage advise always keeping one hand in contact as you work, but if your breaks are smooth, this is not necessary. When working on the floor, in particular, it is better to break contact when you move to a new part of the body, as it is hard to change position without jogging your partner.

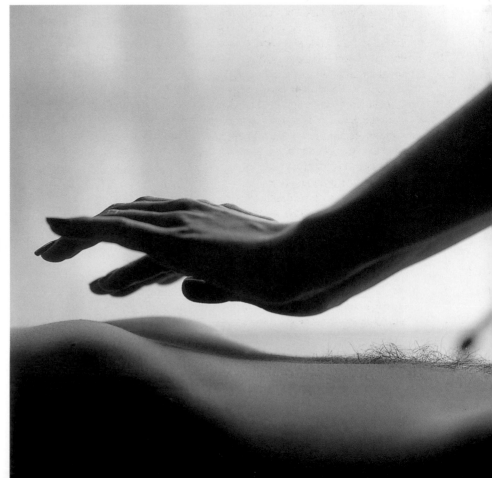

Basic Strokes

A whole body massage consists of a relatively small number of different strokes, repeated in a variety of ways, according to the particular needs of the part you are massaging. For the sake of simplicity, we have divided these strokes into four main types – gliding, medium-depth, deep tissue, and percussion. Professionally, these types are known as effleurage, petrissage, friction, and percussion. Think of them as your ABC of massage with which you can build your own language of touch. When learning new strokes, don't get too preoccupied with matters of technique. It is far more important to stay aware of what you are sensing with your hands and to let your body carry your arms back and forth in a continuous rhythmic dance. Before practising on another person, try the strokes out on your own legs, sitting on the floor. Besides being enjoyable, this will show you how the strokes feel, both from the giver's and the receiver's points of view. Experiment with different speeds and amounts of pressure and, above all, try to develop a sense of rhythm, so that your hands flow from one movement into another, without breaking contact.

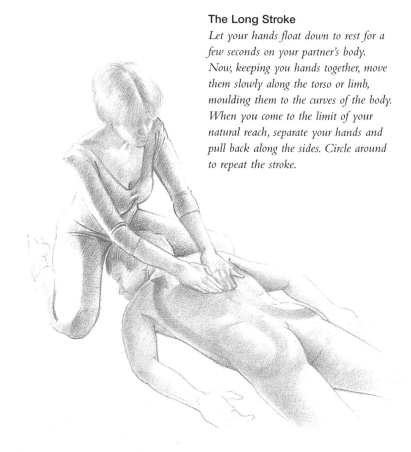

Gliding Strokes (Effleurage)

Like waves rippling over rocks, these gentle rhythmic strokes glide over the skin. By nature general rather than specific, they are used on all parts of the body to begin and end a massage, and as transitional strokes to ease the flow from one movement to another. They never work deeply on the muscle masses. The long stroke is a broad, fluent, and soothing movement. It is used on each part of the body to apply oil and to warm and relax the area. In broad circling, the hands describe large spheres as if doing the breast stroke in miniature. This stroke also serves to spread the oil more evenly over the body. Perform both strokes with your hands relaxed so that their whole surface comes into contact with the receiver's body. Feathering is a brief delicate stroke which brushes over the surface of the skin. It is mainly used to break contact gradually, the strokes fading away like echoes of what has gone before.

The Long Stroke

Let your hands float down to rest for a few seconds on your partner's body. Now, keeping you hands together, move them slowly along the torso or limb, moulding them to the curves of the body. When you come to the limit of your natural reach, separate your hands and pull back along the sides. Circle around to repeat the stroke.

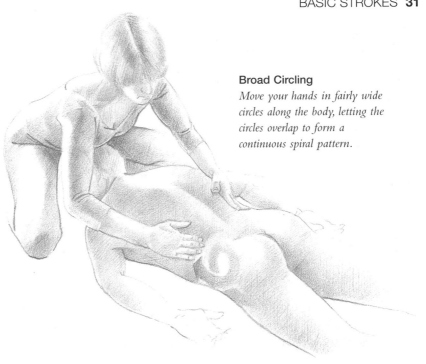

Broad Circling
Move your hands in fairly wide circles along the body, letting the circles overlap to form a continuous spiral pattern.

Feathering *(below)*
Lightly brush your partner's skin with your fingertips, using your hands alternately. Keep your arms and hands relaxed so that you can cover a wide area without changing position.

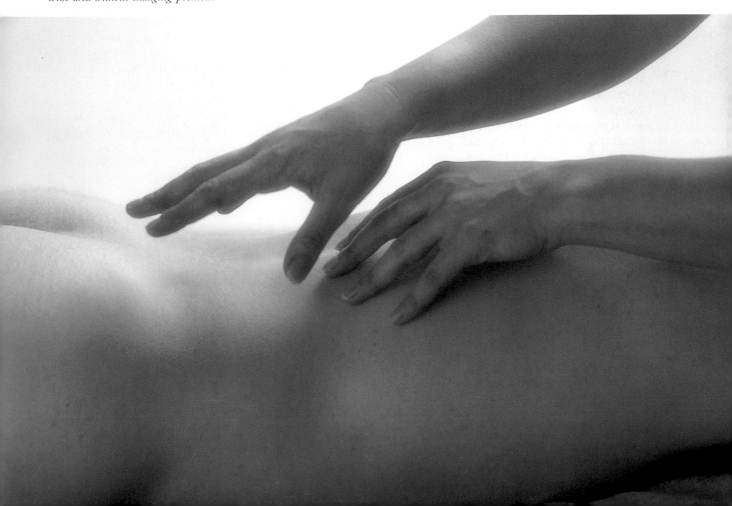

Medium-depth Strokes (Petrissage)

Following on from the gliding strokes, you now start to work more deeply on the large muscle masses, using these kneading, pulling and wringing strokes. In all three, your hands echo one another's movement in a continuously alternating rhythm, relaxing the muscles, draining away waste products, and aiding venous and lymphatic circulation. Kneading consists of alternately squeezing and releasing handfuls of flesh in a broad, circular motion. It is useful for stretching and relaxing the soft, fleshy areas of the body, such as buttocks and thighs. Pulling is a firm lifting stroke used on the sides of the torso and limbs. In wringing, the hands move toward each other from opposite sides, so that the flesh is first bunched up, then stretched between them.

Kneading

Using the whole of your hands, alternately grasp and squeeze bunches of flesh — one hand releasing its hold as the other starts to gather a new handful. Don't lift the hands off the body between strokes; rock smoothly from hand to hand, as if you were kneading dough.

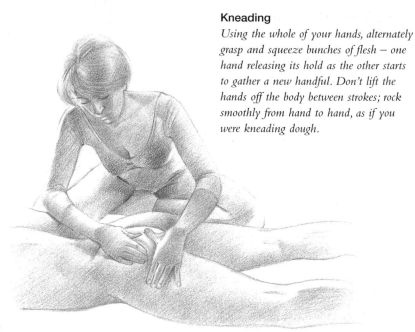

Pulling

Place one hand on your partner's far side, fingertips touching the floor or table and keep the other hand near it. Pull up with alternate hands, each time overlapping the place where the last hand was. Make your movements rhythmical as you slowly work your way along the side.

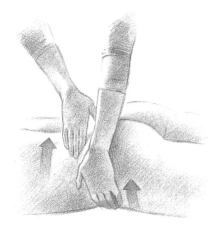

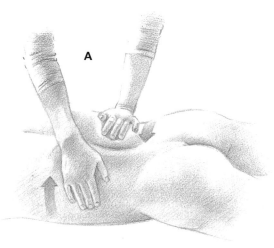

A

Wringing

Place your left hand on your partner's nearest side, heel down, and your right hand on the far side, fingers down. Now push firmly forward with your left hand, and pull back with your right (A). Without stopping, change direction and wring the hands back to the opposite side (B). Move slowly along with each new stroke, keeping the flow continuous.

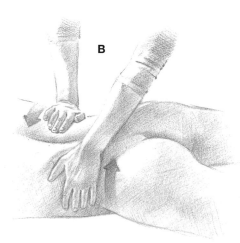

B

Deep Tissue Strokes (Friction)

Deep and focused, these friction movements make use of thumbs, fingertips or heels of hands to reach right down into the tissue to where more hidden tensions may lie. Having soothed and relaxed your partner with the broader, lighter gliding and medium-depth strokes, you now penetrate below the superficial muscle layers or work around the joints with deep tissue strokes. It is important to work deeper gradually. In general, you will find that the body is less fragile than you think, but people vary greatly in their tolerance levels, and although it is sometimes effective to go to the borderline of pain, it is counterproductive to overstep the mark. To perform any of the strokes illustrated, focus your awareness on the parts of the hands you are using, but use your body weight to add depth to your pressure, allowing your hands to remain strong but relaxed.

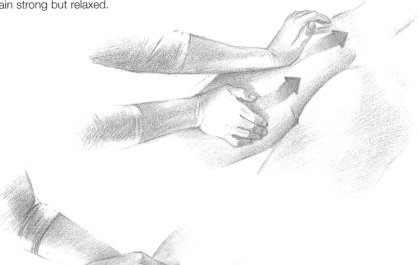

Thumb-rolling
Press the balls of your thumbs away from you into your partner's flesh, using short deep strokes or small circles, depending where you are working. Bring one thumb down just behind the other but push on a little further with each successive stroke so that you eventually cover a fairly broad area.

Heel of Hand Pressure
Push the heels of your hands gently but firmly forward into the flesh, bringing one heel down just behind the other. Let your hands move alternately and rhythmically.

Fingertip Pressure
Using tiny elliptical circles, push in around the joints with your fingertips. Make sure that you are moving the underlying tissue, rather than sliding over the skin surface.

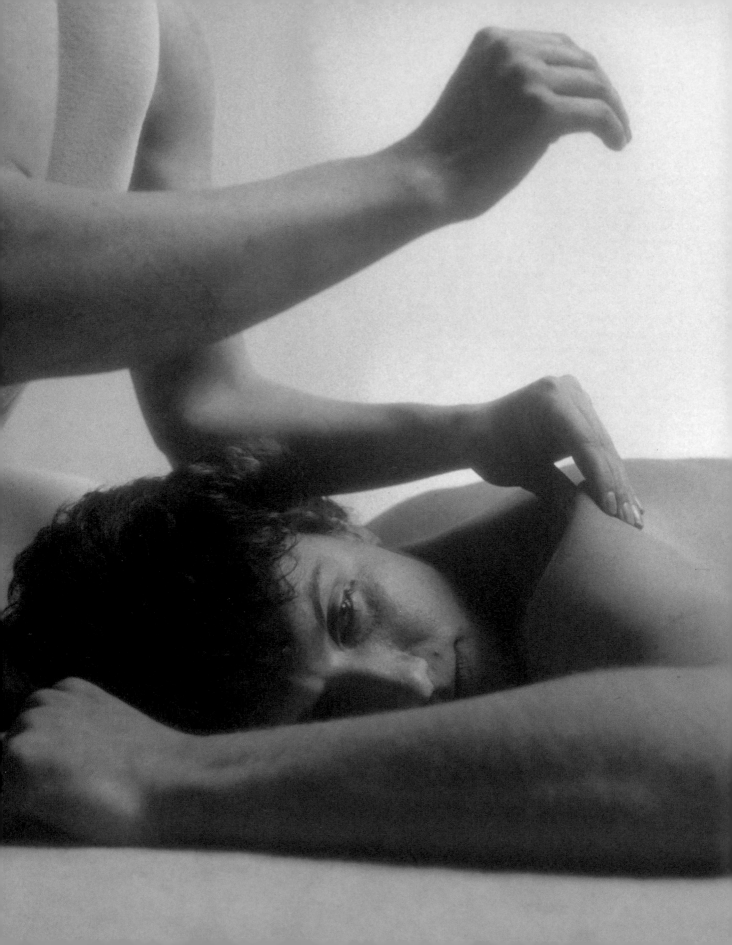

Percussion

Within holistic massage, percussion belongs in a category of its own as, unlike the other strokes, its movements are stimulating rather than relaxing. As its name suggests, it encompasses a range of brisk rhythmic strokes performed repeatedly with alternate hands. Cupping is fairly noisy to apply; hacking, pummelling and plucking are quieter. The main value of percussion is to stimulate the soft-tissue areas, such as thighs and buttocks, toning the skin and improving the circulation. Before trying the strokes out on a partner, practise them on your own leg. Make sure that your hands are relaxed and your wrists loose before you start, and experiment with different speeds and pressures. Percussion is not always appropriate. Reserve it for occasions where a vigorous approach is required.

Hacking

First, shake your hands well to relax them. Now bounce the sides of your hands alternately and fairly rapidly up and down, palms facing one another and fingers loosely together. Wait until you have developed a good rhythm before hacking muscles directly.

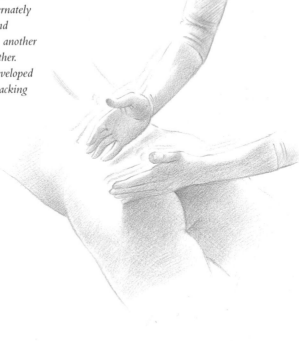

Pummelling

Loosely clench your fists, then repeat the same rhythmic succession of alternate strokes with the fleshy sides of your fists. Let your hands be relaxed so that they bounce firmly yet lightly up and down.

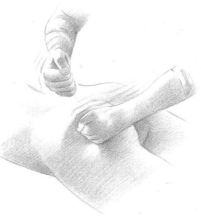

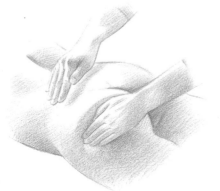

Cupping

Cup your hands, arching them at the knuckles, fingers straight. Now repeat the same rapid sequence of alternate drumming strokes as hacking and pummelling. Your cupped hands trap air against the skin, then release it, making a loud clapping sound.

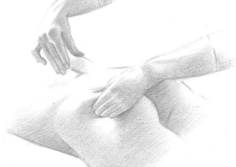

Plucking

Alternately pluck or pinch small bunches of flesh between your thumbs and fingertips. The flesh should slip easily away between the fingers with each plucking stroke.

The Basic Massage Sequence

When learning massage, it will help you to understand and memorize the sequence of strokes if you can see how it is broken down. You start by massaging the back of the body, working down from head to feet, then turn the person over and massage the front of the body, once again working down from the top. The sequence is made up of seven distinct areas – two on the back of the body, five on the front, ending with connecting the whole body. But no matter which area you are working on, you follow roughly the same order of strokes. First you oil the part of the body thoroughly then work from lighter, broader strokes to the deeper, more specific ones, ending once more with lighter ones. When giving a full massage you are affecting many of the body's systems, including the lymphatic and venous circulation, the nervous system, and the "subtle" energies (see pp. 180–9). Traditional massage works "toward the heart", to aid the venous circulation, but since we are interested here in relaxing and balancing a wide range of processes, our sequence of strokes adheres to this rule only where it is particularly appropriate. On the arms and legs, for example, you use firmer strokes toward the heart and lighter ones away from it, to assist the flow of blood back to the heart.

Caution: *There are certain conditions in which massage is contraindicated. These include: skin eruptions, such as boils; infectious skin conditions, such as herpes or scabies; large bruises; varicose veins; fever; areas of swelling or inflammation; recent scar tissue; tumours or any undiagnosed lumps; and cardiovascular problems, such as thrombosis or phlebitis. In these cases you would not work directly over the site of the problem. But you don't have to avoid massage altogether. Gentle work on unaffected areas of the body can be very soothing and comforting. At all times, if you are unsure whether or not massage is appropriate, first check with a doctor.*

1 Back

You start your massage with the back, first working broadly over the whole area, then concentrating on the smaller portions in turn: the shoulderblades and upper back; the lower back, buttocks and sides of the torso; and finally, the spine itself.

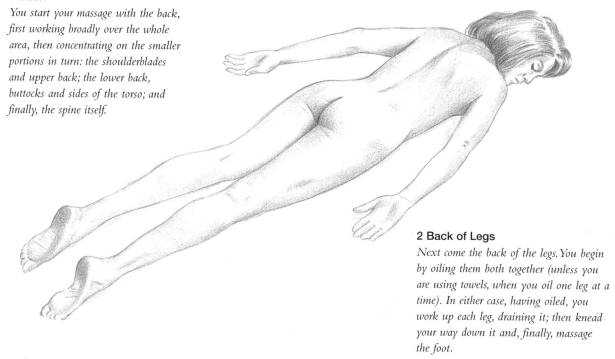

2 Back of Legs

Next come the back of the legs. You begin by oiling them both together (unless you are using towels, when you oil one leg at a time). In either case, having oiled, you work up each leg, draining it; then knead your way down it and, finally, massage the foot.

3 Shoulders, Neck and Scalp

On the front of the body you begin with the shoulders, working on both front and back at once. Next, turning the head to one side you work on each shoulder separately. Then you complete this area by massaging all over the scalp.

4 Face

Here you start at the forehead and travel down to the chin, working outward from the centre to the sides. The eyes, nose, jaw muscles and ears all receive special attention.

5 Arms and Hands

Each arm is massaged separately. As on the leg, you first work up the limb, draining it, then knead down it again, ending by massaging the wrist and hand.

6 Front of Torso

After focusing on the ribcage and sides of the torso, you move down to circle around the abdomen, then work up from the belly in long sweeping strokes.

7 Front of Legs

As for the back of the legs, once you have applied oil, you work up the front of the leg to drain it, circling the kneecap on the way, then knead down the leg again, and end on the foot.

8 Connecting

Finally you link all the parts of the body – either by using long "connecting" strokes or by resting your hands briefly on two separate parts of the body.

Towels and Padding

When receiving a massage, there is nothing more comforting and luxurious than having a soft, warmed towel gently placed over your body. In a professional session, towels are always used to cover the parts of the body not being worked on, for the sake of both privacy and warmth. Practising at home, such elaborate towel technique is generally unnecessary, although partners or friends will often relax more deeply if only half the body is exposed at a time. But it is well worth learning how best to arrange towels, both for occasions when you have a friend who feels shy about remaining uncovered, and when you are massaging someone older or more frail, who may feel the cold more. You will need two bath towels, which you should preferably warm before use by putting them over a radiator. You should also have a smaller hand towel available, to use for women who prefer to have their breasts covered while you massage the front of the torso. Like towels, judiciously placed pillows or cushions add extra comfort and help those receiving massage to relax and let go. They are less important for receivers who are younger or more flexible but, when working with people with lower back problems, support under the knees is essential (see opposite).

The Basic Towel Sequence

Within professional massage, the principle of towel arranging is very simple: you uncover only the part of the client's body that you are going to massage next, leaving the rest covered. And once you have finished working on an area, you cover it once more with a towel. The way you move, arrange, and fold back the towels requires the same sensitivity and awareness you bring to the whole massage, so be sure to avoid throwing them carelessly over the receiver's body or suddenly pulling them off. On these two pages, we show you the precise techniques for neatly covering or uncovering the various areas of the body, following the basic massage sequence. When working at home, just incorporate those techniques that you find most helpful – you don't need to learn and apply them all at this stage.

1 Shoulders and Upper Back

You start by covering the receiver with two towels. Place the lower one vertically down the body, covering the buttocks and legs, and the upper one horizontally across the back and arms. To begin the massage on the shoulders and upper back, simply remove the upper towel, as shown right.

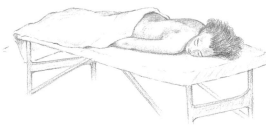

2 Lower Back and Buttocks

Hold the top centre of the lower towel with one hand, using the other hand to fold a triangle of towel back to uncover one buttock and hip. Repeat on the other side, as shown left. This 'paper aeroplane' shape gives access to the lower back and buttocks, without exposing the groove of the buttocks. After completing the whole back and the buttocks, fold the triangles back and replace the upper towel.

Note: *If receivers have kept their underwear on, slide them down carefully beneath the towel, after first asking permission. After massaging the buttocks, pull underwear back up again before working on the legs.*

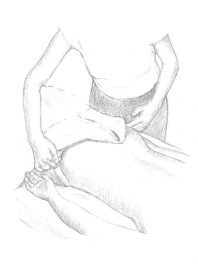

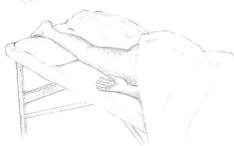

3 Back of Legs

Fold back the bottom corner of the upper towel to uncover one hip and fold the lower towel back over the opposite leg, to expose the whole of one leg and hip. When you have massaged that leg, cover it again and repeat on the other side.

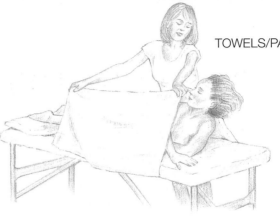

4 Turning

When it's time for the receiver to turn over, it is best to remove the lower towel altogether and anchor the upper towel against the table with your legs. Now reach over to the far side to lift this upper towel at top and bottom, as shown right. Raise it high enough to let the receiver turn over easily without becoming uncovered, and then gently lay it down over the upper body and replace the lower towel.

5 Front of Shoulders and Neck

Fold down the upper towel to reveal the upper chest just above the breasts. Then massage the whole shoulder and neck area. When you come to the face, you can cover the upper chest again, folding the towel over each shoulder for warmth. Leave a little 'collar' of towel around the neck, to avoid pressure on the throat.

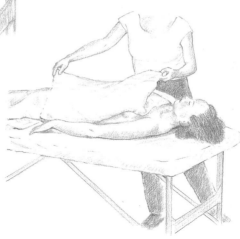

6 Arms

Fold the towel down off the upper chest again and then fold just one side up to cover the shoulder. Next, uncover one arm by folding the towel across the torso, giving you access to the whole arm and shoulder. After massaging, cover it up again and repeat on the other side.

7 Front of Torso and Legs

When working on men, or on women who are comfortable to have their breasts bared, simply remove the upper towel, to massage the front of the torso. Replace the upper towel when you have finished, and then move on to do the legs, uncovering one at a time, as shown for the back of the legs (opposite).

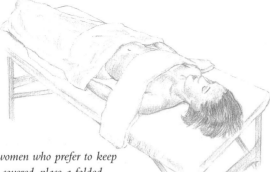

Note: *For women who prefer to keep their breasts covered, place a folded hand towel across the breasts, then gently slide the lower towel away. Adapt your strokes to work separately on the upper chest above the towel and the ribs and abdomen below it.*

Pillows and Cushions

Padding can add greatly to receivers' comfort during a massage, allowing them to sink down and surrender their full weight to the work surface. Before beginning, place a pillow at the foot of the surface, to support the ankles while lying on the front. In cases where the neck is stiff, you may also need a small cushion under the upper chest, to ease strain when the head is turned to one side. And, for those with lower back pain, a pillow under the hips may also be helpful. When the receiver turns over, move the ankle pillow into position beneath the knees, to take the pressure off the lower back. If a person's head tilts back unduly while lying supine, you should also place a folded towel under the head.

The Back

The back is the main supportive structure of the body and an area of great mobility and strength. Since it is more protected than the softer front of the body, it is the best place to start a massage. By the time you come to work on the more vulnerable front of the body, your partner will generally be feeling more trusting and relaxed. The back is also the single largest area you will be massaging and as such it often merits more time and attention than any other part. And because you reach nerves on the back that spread to every part of the body, most people feel a deep sense of release after a thorough back massage. It is imperative that you are comfortable so that you can reach down and across the back easily. To avoid tiring yourself, remember to move your whole body from the hips, rather than using just your arms and shoulders. As your massage begins with the back, it is here that you are accustoming the receiver to your touch and becoming acquainted with the feel of his or her body.

Oiling

To massage the back, lie your partner down on his or her stomach, arms by the sides. Pad under the ankles and, if your partner's neck is a bit stiff, under the upper chest as well. If there is lower back pain, place a pillow under the hips. Now position yourself at your partner's head and spend a few minutes centring yourself before beginning the long oiling stroke. With this stroke you not only spread the oil and warm the back, but you also acquaint yourself with the receiver's body. As you move slowly over the body, shut your eyes and feel the range of sensations beneath your hands – the softness of the skin, the shape of the bones and muscles, the tightness and tension. Let your stroking be an adventure, an exploration.
Note: If using towels, cover the buttocks and legs (see p. 38).

Long Stroke
Bring your hands down gently onto the upper back; then, rocking forward from the hips, begin to travel down the centre, alongside the spinal column. At the base of the spine, let your hands divide and curve around to the sides of the buttocks; then rock back, pulling slowly up the sides, across the shoulders. Repeat until the back is thoroughly oiled.

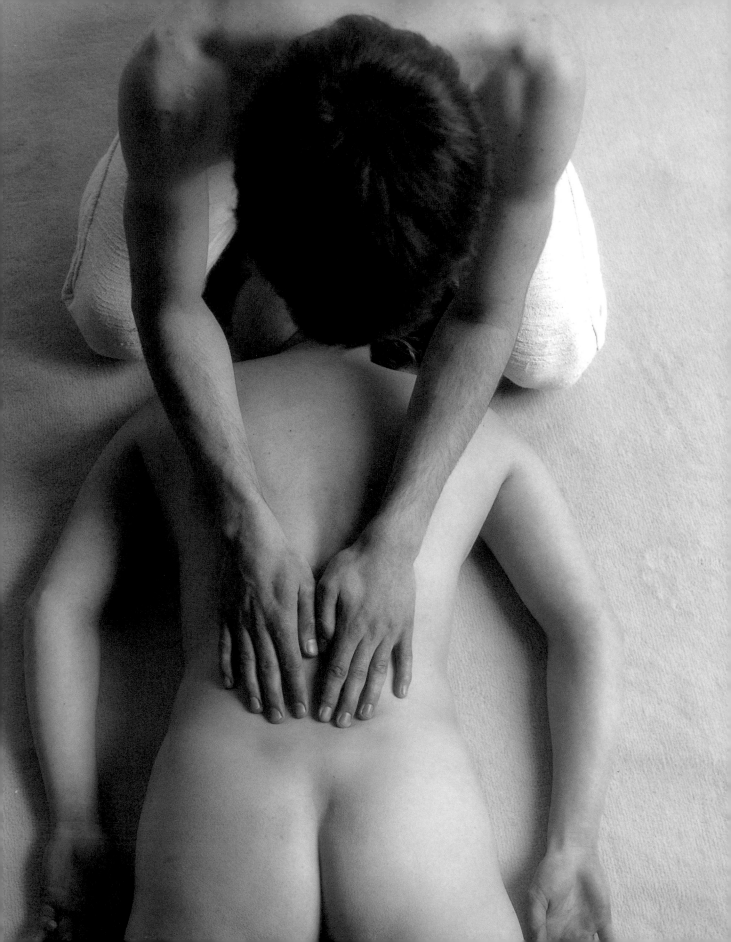

Shoulder from Head

After oiling the back, you start to work on the shoulders, one at a time. Begin with the shoulder away from which the receiver's head is facing. First, circle around the blade and up the side of the ribcage. Then start to work more firmly, kneading all the fleshy areas of the shoulders. Gradually begin to use more pressure, applying the thumb-rolling stroke around the base of the neck and the trapezius muscle (see p. 183). Dwell on any little knots of tension you may find, interspersing this more concentrated work with soothing broader strokes. Finish with deep alternate thumb strokes along the side of the spine.

1 Kneading the Shoulder

Using alternate hands, rhythmically squeeze and gather pockets of flesh. Knead around the blade and along this side of the ribcage, as well as on the shoulder itself, letting your hands follow the contours.

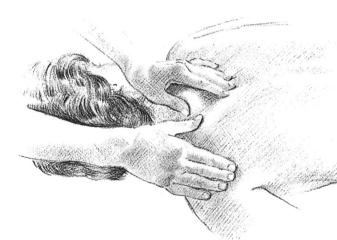

2 Thumb-rolling at Base of Neck

Start to work more deeply with thumb-rolling strokes in the fleshy triangle at the top of the shoulder and the base of your partner's neck. Use small, firm strokes, working increasingly deeply to release any tension. Check that your pressure is acceptable to your partner.

3 Thumbing beside the Spine

Beginning at the base of the neck, push your thumbs alternately along the groove beside the spine in short firm strokes. Travel as far down as the middle of the back, then glide your hands back to the base of the neck and repeat.

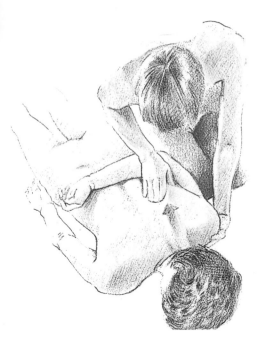

4 Working under the Rim of the Blade

With one hand under the shoulder, use the fingers of the other hand to work around the shoulderblade. Starting at the top of the shoulder, travel slowly down the inner edge of the blade, pushing in firmly as far under the rim as you can. Repeat several times.

Shoulder from Side

You now shift your position to work on the same shoulder from the side, facing your partner's head. Lift the forearm carefully on to the lower back, as shown left. Anchoring the arm on the back, cup your other hand under the shoulder joint – left hand under left shoulder and vice versa. Having isolated the shoulderblade by raising it, use your free hand to begin to work around and across it. Once you have squeezed along the spine of the blade and kneaded the back of the neck, slide your partner's arm down gently off the back and reposition yourself at the head. Help the receiver gently to turn his or her head the other way, when ready, then repeat the sequence on the other shoulder.

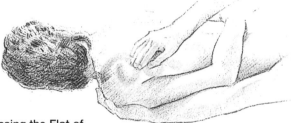

5 Pressing the Flat of the Blade

Now use your fingertips to describe small deep circles on the flat of the blade. Work systematically over the whole area several times.

A

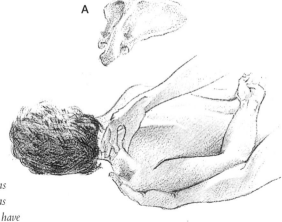

6 Squeezing the Spine of the Blade

The spine of the shoulderblade runs horizontally across its upper half, as shown above right (A). Once you have located it, work along it a few times from the neck outward, squeezing firmly between fingers and thumb.

7 Kneading the Neck

Grasp the muscles at the base of the neck between your fingers and thumb, and squeeze along them. Then firmly knead the neck itself, thoroughly working the whole area.

Repeat 1–7 on the other side.

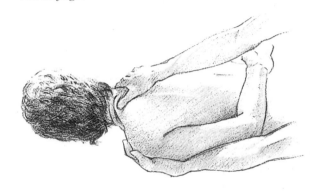

Lower Back and Buttocks

To work on the lower back and buttocks, you must position yourself at your partner's side again, level with the thighs. First you thoroughly knead the lower back; then you massage one buttock, before pulling up that side of the torso. The lower back is a common seat of tension and discomfort. Since it is linked to the *hara* (p. 189), pain in the lumbar region often suggests problems connected with grounding, security and sexuality. A good way of completing the sequence, after pulling up the sides, is to use a gliding stoke down the body from shoulder to foot. Now move to the other side of your partner and repeat the sequence on the opposite buttock and side.

Note: If using towels, bare the lower back and hips (see p. 38).

8 Sacrum and Lumbar Circling

With alternate hands, circle around the sacrum and lumbar spine using a flat kneading stroke. Move quite broadly over the whole area, rocking your pelvis from side to side as you circle.

9 Kneading the Buttocks *(below)*

Move your hands down to the buttock furthest away from you and begin to knead deeply, gathering parcels of flesh in one hand after the other. Work around the entire buttock, as you squeeze and wring.

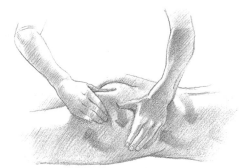

10 Plucking the Buttocks

Using alternate hands, pick up small pockets of flesh between thumb and fingers. Try to maintain a fairly rapid but regular rhythm, and keep your hands relaxed and your wrists loose.

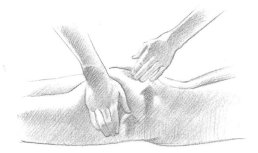

11 Pulling up the Sides

Starting at the buttocks, use alternate hands to pull steadily up the far side of the body. Make sure there is always one hand in contact with the body.

Repeat 9–11 on the other side.

Spine

According to yoga, the condition of the spine affects us at every level – physical, emotional, and spiritual. The spinal nerves link the brain with all the other parts of the body and since they lie close to the surface of the back, massage can have a profoundly relaxing effect. Spinal massage divides into three main strokes: a broad stroke, called the "rocking horse", which is in two parts, one soothing, the other more stimulating; a deep friction stroke which eases tension around the vertebrae; and finally, a connecting stroke with your forearms which imparts a feeling of wholeness to the entire back. In general, you avoid pressing directly on the vertebrae and work on either side of the spine, letting you hands melt away any knots you find as you work up the back.

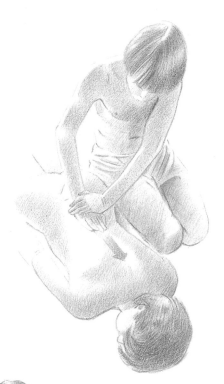

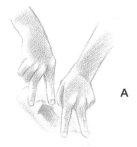

A

12 "Rocking Horse"

Rest one hand on top of the other and glide both firmly up from the base of the spine to the neck. Using your index and middle fingertips (A) press down on either side of the spine, with one hand overlapping the path of the other, so that you ripple gradually down along the whole spine and off at the coccyx.

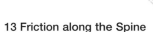

13 Friction along the Spine

Make short deep circles with your thumbs up either side of the spine. Press them briefly into the hollows at the base of the skull, before sweeping lightly back down.

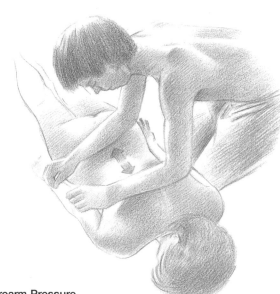

14 Forearm Pressure

Place your inner forearms in the centre of your partner's back. Slowly pull them apart, bringing one up to the neck, the other to the base of the spine. Repeat, working diagonally across the back, so that one arm goes over one shoulder, the other off the opposite buttock. Repeat, crossing diagonally in the opposite direction.

Back of Legs

To complete your massage on the back of the body you work on the legs, and finally on the feet. In bringing energy down to the legs and feet, you are helping your partner to feel more grounded and stable. The soft, fleshy backs of the legs are ideal for kneading and wringing. If this area is especially sensitive or painful, you may find that your partner suffers from lower back problems, since the sciatic nerve runs from the base of the spine right down the back of the leg to the heel. By massaging the back of the leg you therefore not only relieve tenderness there but also affect pain or stiffness in the lower back.

Caution: *Avoid all but gentle strokes up the leg if your partner has varicose veins. Deep massage might aggravate the condition. Work on either side of the veins and don't stroke down the legs at all.*

Oiling

Place yourself between your partner's feet and start by oiling both legs at once, one hand on each leg. If you are working from a kneeling position, rock forward from the hips as you glide up the legs. Now choose which leg you are going to work on first and position yourself at the foot. To spread the oil thoroughly and warm the leg before massage, you can either use the long stroke with your fingers pointing straight up the leg, or cup your hands, as shown right.
Note: If using towels, uncover and oil one leg at a time (see p. 38).

Cupped Hand Stroke

Cup your hands over the back of the ankle (A), with the left hand above the right, if working on the left leg, and vice versa. Glide both hands up the middle of the back of the leg. When you near the top, allow the leading hand to go up over the buttock and around the hip joint while the other moves around to the inside thigh (B). Glide both hands down the sides of the leg and off the foot (C). Take care not to get too close to the genitals when pulling down the inside thigh. Respect your partner's privacy at all times.

Long Stroke on Both Legs *(below)*
Oil your hands and let them rest for a moment on the backs of the ankles. Now glide your hands up the centre of your partner's legs – over the buttocks and round the hips, sliding down along the sides of the legs, over the sides of the feet and off the toes. Repeat once or twice.

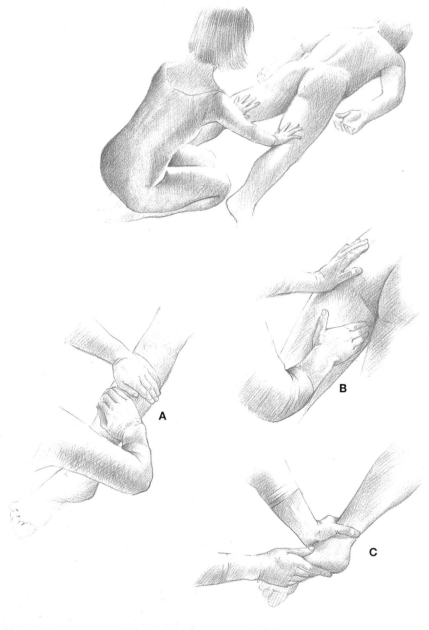

A

B

C

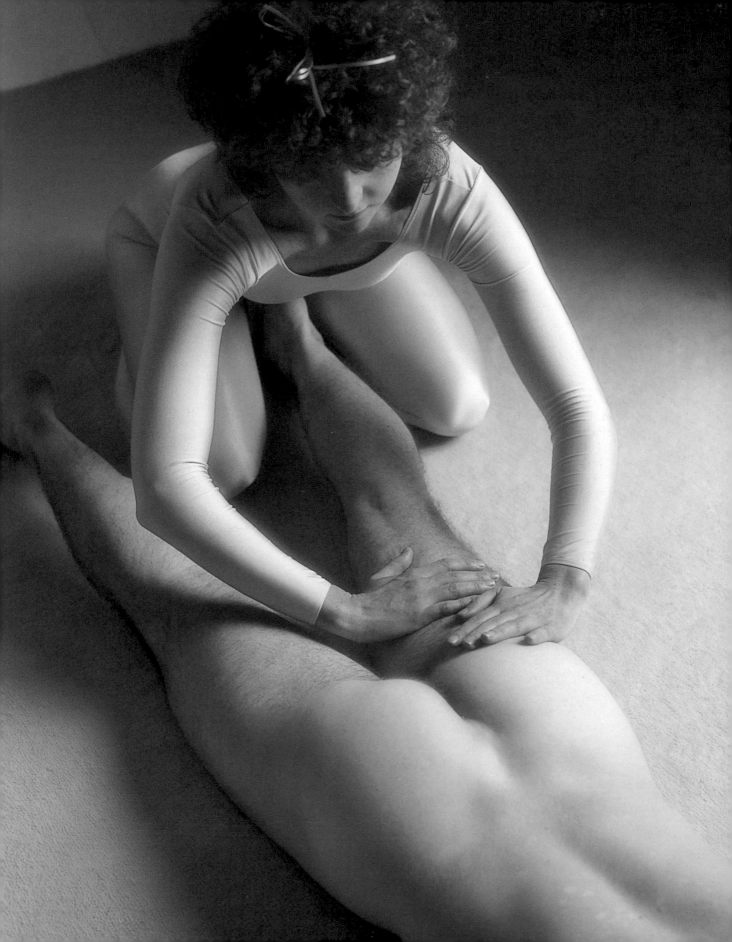

"Half Locust" Leg Lift

In addition to using the different strokes to massage your partner, you can incorporate various "passive" exercises into your session. These mobilize the joints and stretch the muscles by placing the receiver's body in certain positions. The "Half Locust" Leg Lift – so-called because the movement imitates the Half Locust position in yoga – is useful during leg massage as it exercises the hip joint and stretches the muscles at the front of the thigh. When lifting your partner's leg, let your whole body take the weight, not just your shoulders and arms. And flex the leg only as far as the point of resistance. There should be no strain or discomfort, either for you or the receiver.

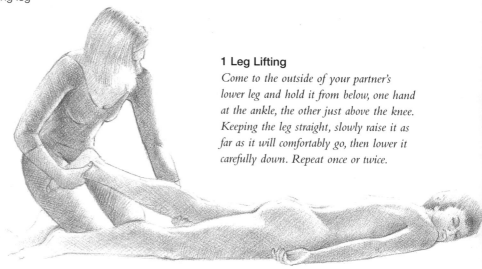

1 Leg Lifting

Come to the outside of your partner's lower leg and hold it from below, one hand at the ankle, the other just above the knee. Keeping the leg straight, slowly raise it as far as it will comfortably go, then lower it carefully down. Repeat once or twice.

Draining the Leg

These strokes work with the circulation, assisting the flow of blood back to the heart. Positioned either at your partner's foot or by the side of the leg, you begin to work up from the ankle, first with your thumbs, then with the heels of your hands. When you come to the back of the knee, your strokes should be broader and lighter – if you press too hard, the kneecap will be pushed uncomfortably against the working surface. The draining stroke with the heels of the hands is most effective on the back of the thigh and buttocks, where there is a generous expanse of flesh, but you can also use it on the calves.

2 Draining with Thumbs

Working just below the calf, use alternate thumbs to press gradually up the calf and thigh in short firm strokes. Keep the rest of your hand in contact with the leg, to "anchor" your thumbs.

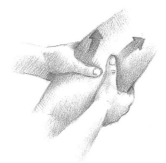

3 Draining with Heels of Hands

Work slowly up the leg, pressing the heels of your hands into it alternately in broad, deep strokes. Let your movement be continuous and rhythmic and relax your hands.

Working down the Leg

Having drained the leg up to the hip, you now begin to move down again toward the foot, using a kneading stroke on the thigh and calf. After thoroughly massaging the entire leg, you can either pull down the inside of the leg in overlapping strokes or wring your hands along the leg (see p. 32). The back of the leg is particularly suitable for wringing work as there are no protruding bones to interrupt your path.

4 Kneading the Leg
Using a rhythmical alternating movement between your two hands, gather and squeeze bunches of flesh over the whole of the thigh and calf. Maintain close contact with the leg – you don't need to lift your hands into the air between handfuls.

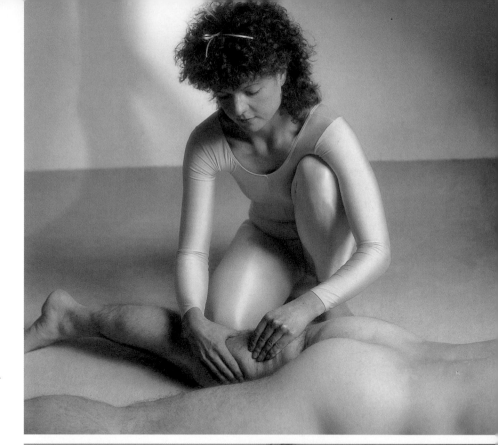

5 Wringing along the Leg
Starting at the lower calf, wring your hands gradually up and then down the back of the leg. Keep your pressure even.

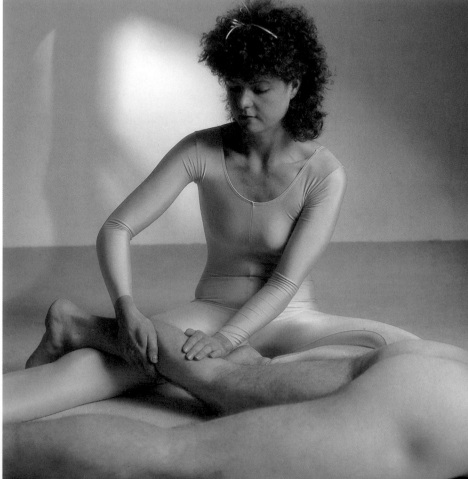

The Ankle

Like any other joints, ankles often store tension, blocking the free flow of energy between the feet and the legs. People with stiff ankles may suffer from cold feet and may be "ungrounded" (see p. 170), so that their connection with the ground, with reality, is unsure. Massage will not only help to restore flexibility and assist grounding and energy flow, it will also relieve any build-up of fluid. The movements shown here serve both to test and then to increase mobility and suppleness in this area. Rotating the ankle gives you a sense of the flexibility of the joint; flexing the foot tests the tension in the muscles and tendons. If the hamstrings are tight, you will not be able to push the foot far forward; if the extensor muscles at the front of the lower leg are tight, pushing the foot backward will be painful.

Lifting the Lower Leg

In order to work on the ankles and feet, you first need to lift the lower leg. Positioned beside your partner's leg, place one hand under the ankle and the other on the back of the knee. Slowly lift the lower leg to an upright position. Notice whether your partner "helps" by raising the leg or readily surrenders the leg to you.

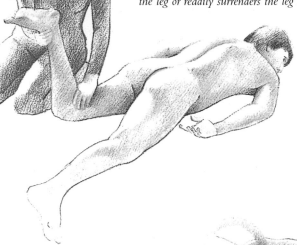

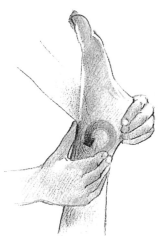

6 Working around the Ankle

Holding the foot firmly with one hand, use the other to work around the ankle bone with fingers or thumb. Loosen around the joint with small circling strokes, first on one side of the leg and then on the other.

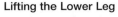

7 Rotating the Ankle

Holding the leg just above the ankle with one hand, grasp the foot with the other and slowly move it around in a wide circle, first in one direction for a few turns, then in the opposite direction. Circle the foot to the limits of its flexibility.

8 Pushing the Foot Down and Up

Grasp the ankle with one hand and push down on the toes and ball of the foot with the other, flexing the foot as far as its resistance point (A). Then pull the front of the foot backward with one hand and push down on the heel with the other, stretching the top of the foot and the front of the leg (B).

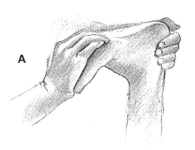

A

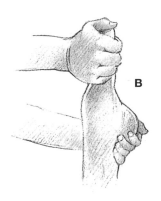

B

The Foot

The human foot has evolved into a highly complex structure, made up of 26 small bones, some of which form two large supporting arches. As well as carrying the entire weight of the body, feet serve as marvellous shock absorbers. In addition, the sole of the foot contains thousands of nerve endings with reflex connections to the whole of the rest of the body (see pp. 136–7). In massaging the feet, therefore, you are affecting the entire body, not just the feet themselves. For this reason, many masseurs concentrate on a foot massage when there is not enough time for a full body massage. Once you have finished one foot, lower the leg carefully back down, then move over to work on the back of the other leg and foot, starting from the beginning of the sequence. Treating the feet ends the massage on the back of the body. After completing both legs let your partner rest for a few moments. Then suggest that he or she turns gently over, ready to receive massage on the front of the body. **Note:** If using towels, hold them up while the receiver turns over (see p. 39).

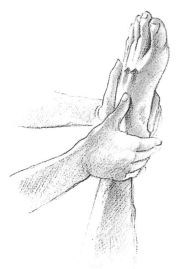

9 Cleaning between the Tendons
With one hand, hold the sole of the foot, toes pointing upward. Use the thumb or fingers of the other hand to press slowly along each channel between the tendons from toes to ankle.

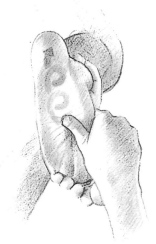

10 Thumbing the Sole
Supporting the foot with one hand, work across the whole of the sole with the thumb of the other hand, making small, firm circling strokes. It is best to start at the heel and end at the ball of the foot, just under the toes.

11 Stretching the Toes
Working systematically along the toes, first stretch them apart sideways, then stretch each toe backward and forward. Be sure to check how far you can stretch the toes with your partner – it is often farther than you imagine.

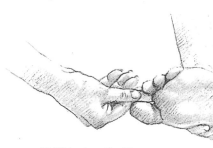

12 Wringing the Toes
One at a time, hold each toe at the base between your thumb and fingers and tug steadily, twisting it a little from side to side as your fingers slide to the tip and off. As you come off each toe, shake your hand, ridding yourself of any negative energy.

Repeat oiling and strokes 1–12 on the other leg.

Shoulders, Neck, and Scalp

Once your partner has turned over, you begin your massage on the front of the body by returning to the shoulders, one of the principal storehouses of tension in the body. In a healthy individual, feelings that arise at gut level are expressed physically through the arms and hands, or vocally, through the throat. But many of us are forbidden to express our emotions freely as children, and learn to suppress feelings of anger or sorrow by tightening up in the shoulders and throat. So this area merits special attention from both the back and front of the body. The main advantage of working on the shoulders from the front is that the receiver's own weight presses down on to your hands under the back, giving extra impact to the strokes. The sequence of strokes may seem a little complex at first, as a lot of it happens out of sight, between your partner's back and the working surface. But once you have learnt it, you will find it a most rewarding part of your massage session, and one that feels especially good to the receiver.

Long Stroke
A *Place your hands on the upper chest just below the collarbone, fingers pointing toward one another. Slowly draw them apart, heels leading out toward the shoulders.*

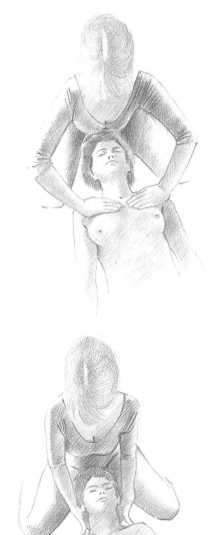

B *As you reach the shoulders, curve your hands round the joints, then slide them along the tops of the shoulders, until you come to the back of the neck.*

Oiling
Once your partner has turned over, move the ankle pillow to beneath the knees, and check if he or she needs a small folded towel under the head (see p. 39). Then sit down at the head end and begin to apply oil in one continuous long stroke to the whole upper chest, shoulder, and neck area, as described in the three steps shown here. If you are following the whole massage sequence, your partner's upper back will already be oily. But if you wish to treat this part in isolation, you should oil the whole upper back before your partner lies down.
Note: If using towels, fold the top one down, as shown on page 39.

C *Continue the stroke up the back of the neck to the base of the skull, then up the back of the head and off the crown. Repeat the whole stroke a few times.*

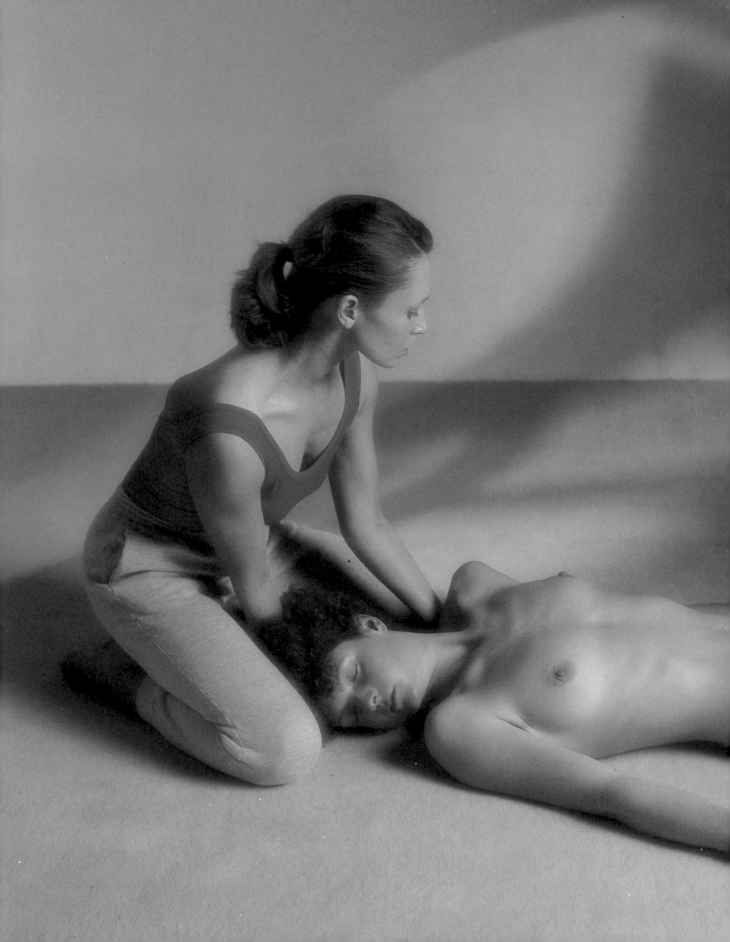

Neck Stretches

These stretching movements lead on naturally from the long stroke. Instead of bringing your hands off the top of the head, you simply stop at the base of the skull and, holding the head securely, rock your body backward to stretch the neck. You can also stretch the neck forward, backward, and to one side. This stretches right along the top of the shoulder and side of the neck. Many people will be relaxed enough to surrender their heads to your hands – their heads will feel heavy when you lift them. Others who are tense will unconsciously move their heads themselves. If this happens, simply ask your partner to be aware that they are "holding on" while you attempt to loosen the neck by stretching it. But don't be impatient if they are unable to "let go". Just carry on to the next stroke.

1 Stretching the Neck

Cup both hands firmly under the head, fingers at the base of the skull. Lift the head a little way off the work surface and rock backward, so that you stretch the back of the neck. Lower the head gently.

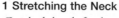
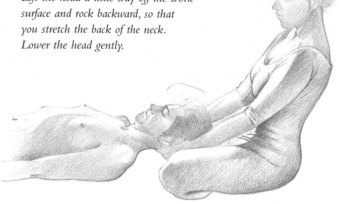

2 Stretching the Neck Up and Down

With your hands still cupped under the head, lift the head up and bring the chin toward the chest, as shown left. Slowly bring the head back again and this time move one hand down to the nape and lift the neck, letting the head tilt right back, as shown below. Now straighten the neck again.

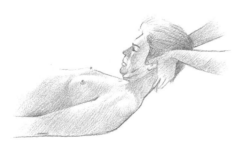

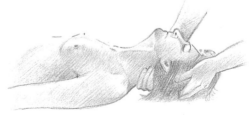

3 Stretching the Neck from Side to Side

Holding the back of the head securely in one hand, "carry" it slowly toward one shoulder while pressing down on the opposite shoulder with the other hand. Bring the head back to the centre, reverse your hands and repeat on the other side.

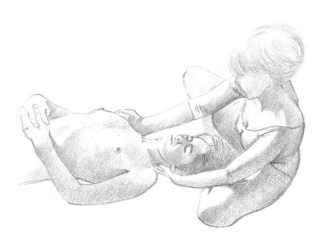

Shoulder, Front, and Back Sequence

Now you have loosened the whole neck up a little, you start to focus on one side at a time. Laying the head on its side on one hand, you use the other hand to work the whole upper back and neck area on the opposite side, using the three-part sequence shown below. Since much of the sequence takes place out of sight, under the back, we have provided diagrams to illustrate the path of your hands. The sequence consists of pushing your hand under the back, then pulling up toward the neck across three different areas of the back in a fan shape. You will find it easier to get your hands under some backs than others. Don't try too hard – be content to go as far as you can comfortably manage, without stress. As you pull your hand toward you, the flesh may bunch up at the neck. If this happens, don't try to hop over it – just carry on slowly up and your pressure will gradually release the folds. It is important that you execute this sequence of strokes slowly and with awareness.

Turning the Head

Hold the head on either side, thumbs just above the ears, fingers behind them. Lift the head slightly and gently turn it to rest on one cupped hand. Check that you are not pulling any hair and that your partner's head is comfortable. You begin by working on the shoulder away from which your partner is facing.

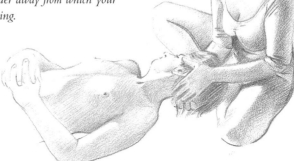

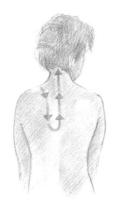

4 Shoulder, Front, and Back Sequence

A *Begin the sequence as for the long stroke (p. 52), but instead of going up the neck push down alongside the spine, as far as you can comfortably. Then pull your curved fingers very slowly up the groove at the side of the spine and up the back of the neck to the base of the skull. Now use your fingers to make tiny arches all along this side of the base of the skull, working just under the rim of the bone. Repeat once more.*

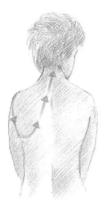

B *Begin as before, but when your hand reaches the shoulder joint, curve your fingers round under the shoulder and push down along your partner's side. When you reach the waist pull diagonally across the back and shoulderblade, with fingers slightly curved, until you come back to the neck and base of the skull. After circling as before at the base of the skull, repeat the movement a couple of times.*

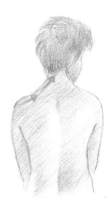

C *Begin as before, but once your hand has circled the shoulder joint pull along the top of the shoulders and up the side and back of the neck with your thumb over the front of the shoulder and your fingers behind. The inside edge of the index finger and the web of the thumb should create a taut band. After circling as before at the base of the skull, repeat the stroke. Then leave your partner's head in your hand to work on the scalp (p. 56).*

The Scalp

Surprisingly, the scalp can get tense and contribute to tension headaches and also to hair problems, such as dandruff and hair loss. Massage helps to relieve this tightness and aids the circulation; in the process it also improves the health of the hair. Once you have completed the three strokes shown here, cup your free hand over your partner's ear and very gently turn the head to the other side.

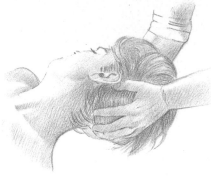

5 Rotating the Scalp

Spread your hand over the head and rotate it, moving the scalp against the bone, as shown left.

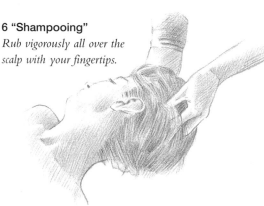

6 "Shampooing"

Rub vigorously all over the scalp with your fingertips.

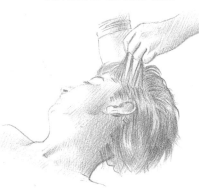

7 "Pulling off" the Hair

Taking a bunch of hair at a time, pull from the roots and slowly slide your fingers off.

Repeat 4–7 on the other side.

Spinal Stretch

This is the only stroke in the Front of Shoulders and Neck sequence that requires cooperation on the part of the receiver, who must lift up his or her back to enable you to reach under it with your hands. The stroke provides the whole spine with a wonderful stretch and feels remarkably good to the receiver. You may need to practise a little before you can execute it really smoothly. But you should be able to manage it, unless your partner is very heavy or much larger than yourself – in which case omit it from the sequence. Be sure to always pull from the *hara* and pelvis, not just from the shoulders. Repeat the stretch once or twice if you are comfortable with it.

8 Spinal Stretch

Ask your partner to arch his or her back a little so that you can push your hands as far under it as possible, placing your palms up alongside the spine (A). Now ask your partner to relax on to your arms. Once you feel that they have fully "let go", start to rock your body backward, pulling your hands up along the grooves beside the spine, fingertips curved up a little (B). Travel very slowly along the whole length of the spine, up the neck and back of the head (C) and end by "pulling off" the hair.

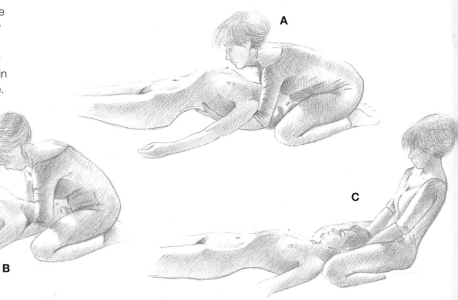

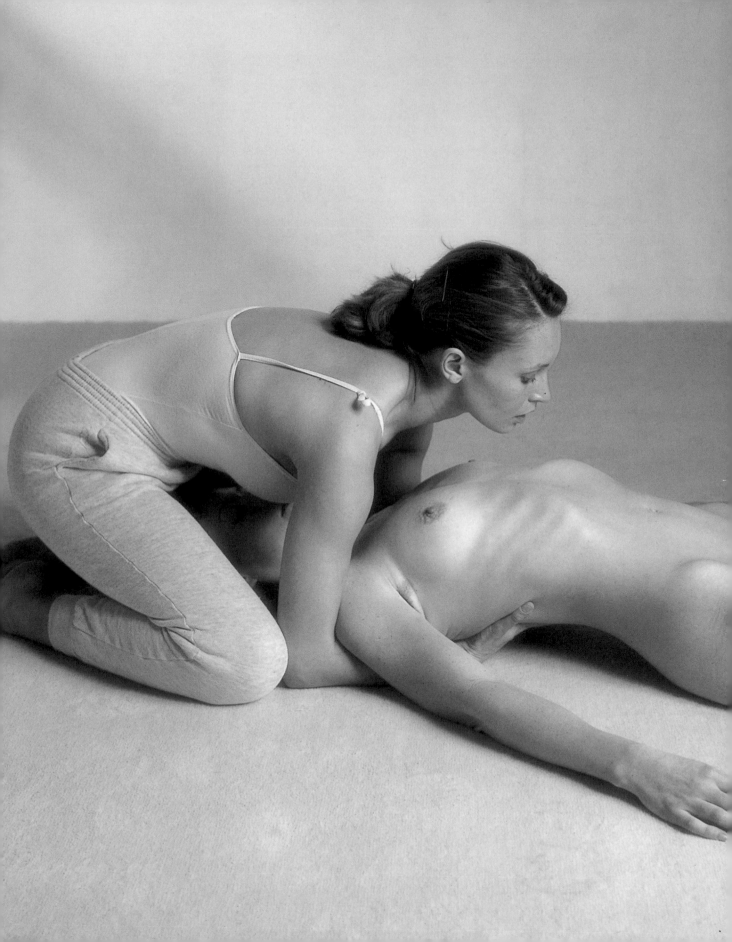

The Face

The face is generally the part we notice first in other people. It is uncovered, exposed, and belies the history of its owner, whether openly or secretly. Its expression is sculpted by the myriad of tiny muscles that give us the mobility to make faces. Stress and tension are reflected in tightness around the brow, jaw and eyes, joy and serenity in an open relaxed expression. And whether we wear a constantly smiling mask of appeasement or one of mock surprise, with eyebrows fixedly raised, the patterns frozen on our faces help reveal our attitudes and character. By enabling us to relinquish some of our masks, a caring face massage can lead to a sense of deep relaxation and "connectedness" throughout the whole body, and to the comfort of just enjoying "being", without having to appear to be something else. If there is not time to do a full body massage, you might consider just doing the face as, like the feet, the face mirrors other parts of the body (see p. 177).

The Face

You may not need to oil your hands to massage the face, as what you already have on your fingers may be enough for this relatively small area. Before giving a face massage for the first time, practise on your own face to see how it feels. The face is bonier and less fragile than it looks and you may be surprised to find that you can apply quite deep pressure without discomfort. Thresholds of comfort vary, however, so you should be sure to get feedback from your partner. Before beginning, check whether your partner is wearing contact lenses; if so, refrain from working over the eyelids. In this sequence, you work gradually down the face, stroking across it in strips from the centre to the sides. Make your movements slow and "clean" and keep your awareness in your fingers. Since many of the strokes on the face are quite small, you need to take care to avoid overtensing your shoulders. Even the smallest strokes benefit from rocking back and forth from the hips.

Position for Working on Face
You remain sitting or standing at your partner's head for the whole of this sequence. Keep your pressure even as you work down from forehead to chin.

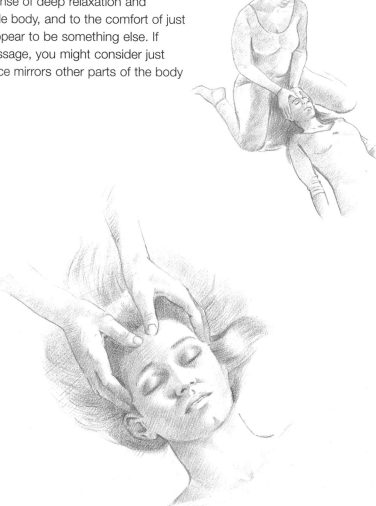

1 Forehead
Place your thumbs at the centre of the forehead, just above the brows, anchoring your hands on the sides of the head. Moving up a strip at a time, draw your thumbs apart slowly, coming out over the hair and off the sides of the head. Cover the whole forehead in this way, travelling up as far as the hairline.

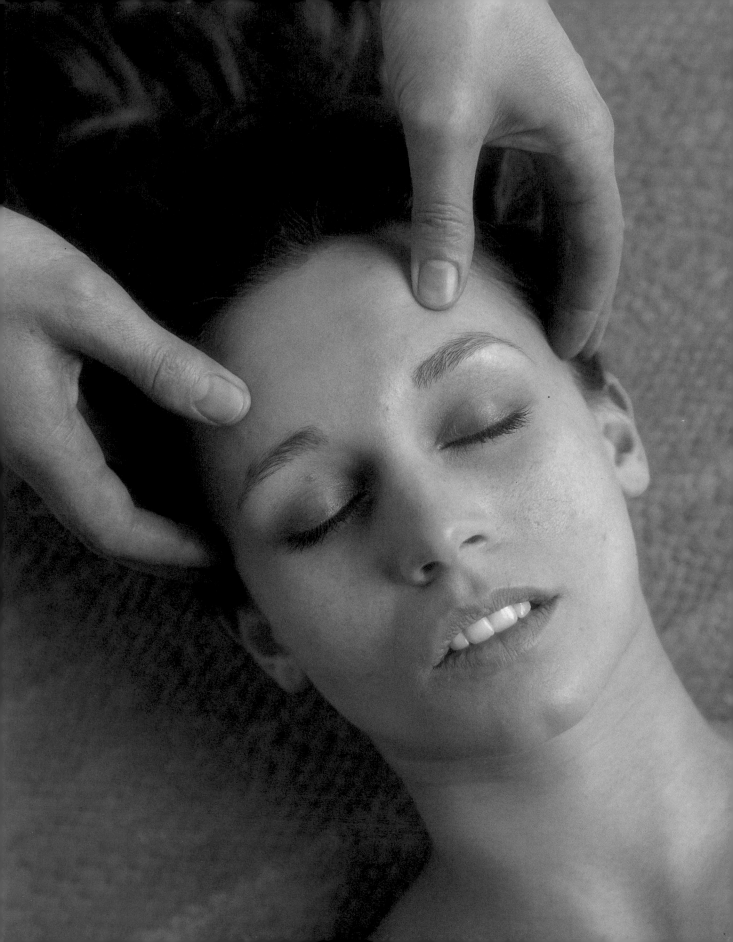

Eyes, Nose and Cheeks

Continuing on down the face, you now work over the eyebrows, eyelids, and nose to the chin. Twelve pairs of cranial nerves link the brain directly with the face and the five senses. Working around the eyes, eyebrows, and temples in particular, often helps enormously to soothe away stress, relieve headaches and clear the sinuses.

2 Eyebrows

Starting at the inner end of the eyebrows, draw your thumbs firmly out to the sides over the hairline and off the head, smoothing the entire browline. Repeat four times.

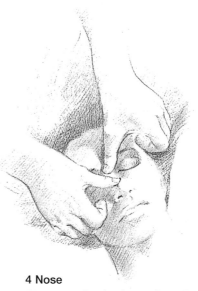

3 Eyes

Draw your thumbs smoothly and gently over the eyelids, from the inner to the outer corners and off the sides of the head. Repeat once or twice.

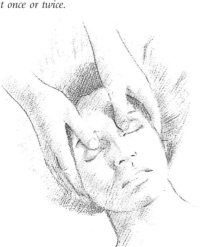

4 Nose

Using your thumbs alternately, stroke down the bridge of the nose from the top to the tip. Then squeeze the tip of the nose gently between your thumbs and index fingers.

5 Cheeks

Beginning just under the inner corner of the eyes, stroke your thumbs across the cheekbone to the hairline above the ear and off the head. Repeat the stroke in strips as you travel gradually down the face — below the cheekbone, above the upper lip and below the lower one. When working near the nose, be careful not to close the breathing passages.

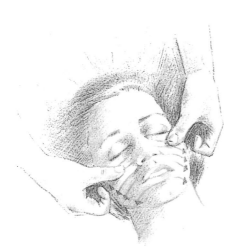

Chin and Jawline

Massaging the lower part of the face consists of squeezing the chin, working along the jawbone and then circling over the chewing muscles, or masseters. If you find it hard to locate these muscles, place your fingers on the cheeks and ask your partner to clench their teeth. You will feel the muscles rise up and harden as they contract. In the face map (p. 177) the jaw is related to the pelvis, and tension in one usually means tension in the other. If your partner holds a lot of tension in the hips, it is often helpful to loosen the jaw before working directly on the pelvis.

6 Chin
Hold the point of the chin between your thumbs and index fingers and squeeze along the whole chin, using a rhythmical "milking" stroke.

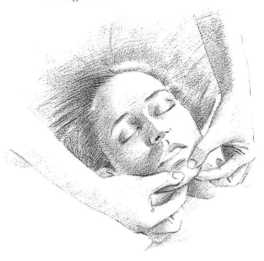

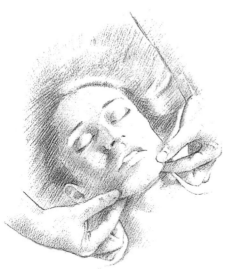

7 Jawbone
Hold the rim of the jawbone at the chin, then draw your hands slowly apart, squeezing right along the jawbone as far as the ear lobe.

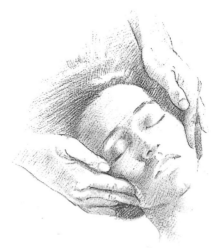

8 Chewing Muscles
Locate the chewing muscles on each side of the face. Then circle slowly over them with the flats of your fingers.

Cheeks and Ears

This two-part sequence begins with a broad stroke across the cheeks and ends with stretching and squeezing the ears. Way back in our history we were able to move our ears – some people still retain the ability to wiggle them. The ears contain acupuncture points for each part of the body. This may explain why it is so pleasurable to have your ears massaged.

9 Cheek to Ear Stroke

A *Put the heels of your hands on either side on the nose, with your fingers pointing toward the ears. Now slowly part your hands, gliding them firmly over the cheeks toward the ears.*

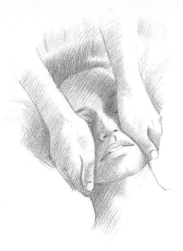

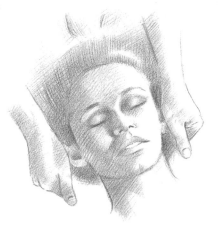

B *Grasp the ears between your fingers and the heels of your hands and very gently stretch them away from the head. Then squeeze all around them with your fingers and thumbs.*

Connecting the Face and the Head

This is a long stroke in three parts, connecting the face with the neck and head. For best effect, let it be one smooth flowing movement, ending in a gentle stretching of the neck. You can repeat the stroke several times then finish if you wish by resting one hand lightly on the forehead and the other on the upper chest to connect head and body. After holding it for a moment or two, softly break contact.

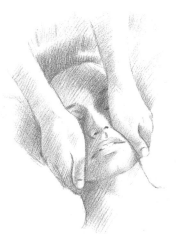

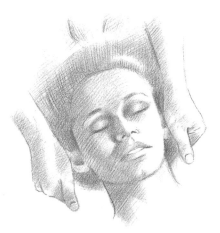

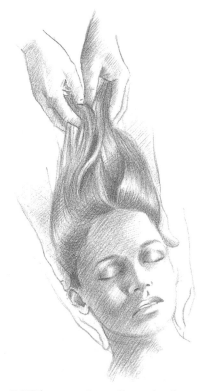

10 Connecting the Face and the Head

A *Cup your palms over your partner's eyes with your thumbs on either side of the nose. Remain there for a moment, allowing the eyes to rest within the darkness of your hands.*

B *Fingers first, begin to slide your hands smoothly down over the face, across cheeks and under the ears to the back of the neck.*

C *Without stopping, pull your hands up the neck and, cupping your hands under the back of the head, draw them toward you coming slowly off the top of the head and then the hair.*

Arms and Hands

When we evolved from walking on four legs and stood upright, we freed our upper limbs for a variety of uses – to get food and fuel and to ward off danger, for example. We also exposed our soft bellies, and our relationships with each other acquired a new sensitivity. The arms and hands are intimately connected to relating – how we relate to each other and to the world at large, how we give and take. They are instruments of doing and expressing – out of which feelings can flow freely, provided no chronic tensions are present in the shoulder and throat area (see p. 175). Through our arms and hands, we express our most powerful emotions, showing love by embracing, giving, protecting, or stroking, and hatred or rage through hitting, punching, or shaking our fists. An arm and hand massage is thus a marvellously liberating and relaxing experience, especially for those who tend to "bottle up" their feelings.

Long Stroke
A *Rest your oiled hands on your partner's wrist, fingers pointing up the arm. Now glide your hands up the arm, undulating over the contours, as shown below.*

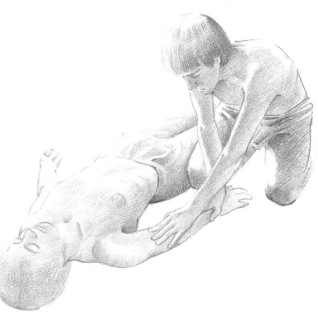

Oiling

To work on the arms and hands, you move to your partner's side, level with the hips and facing the head. As usual you start by oiling and warming one of the arms, using the long stroke. Always keep these initial strokes slow. Help your partner to become aware of each new part of the body gradually so that they can enjoy rediscovering their bodies without feeling bombarded. For the sake of clarity, the long stroke, right, is presented in two steps, although it is executed as one continuous stroke. You should repeat the whole stroke once or twice. As a variation you can also oil the arms with cupped hands, as shown on page 46.
Note: If using towels, bare one arm at a time, as shown on page 39.

B *Just before you reach the shoulder joint, let your leading, or "outside", hand curve over the joint, while your other hand curves down on to the inner arm, just below the armpit, as shown above. Embracing as much of the arm as possible, pull your hands down the arm to the wrist. Enfold your partner's hand in your two palms as you slide them down and off the fingertips.*

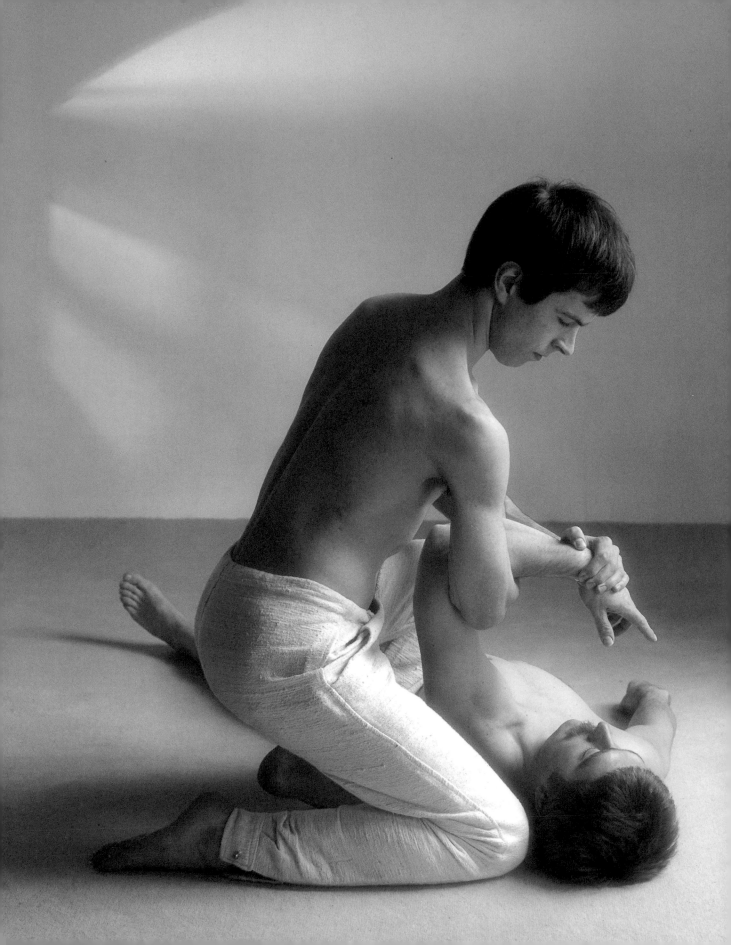

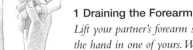

Draining the Arm

This sequence works with the circulation of blood and lymph in the arm. Its purpose is to assist the lymphatic flow and the blood's venous return to the heart. Veins are closer to the skin's surface than arteries, which carry blood away from the heart. They therefore respond more readily to external pressure. You start by draining the forearm, then work systematically along the upper arm. While squeezing down the forearm, you may notice your partner's fingers opening and closing. This is because the muscles controlling the fingers are in the forearm.

1 Draining the Forearm

Lift your partner's forearm slightly and hold the hand in one of yours. With your other hand hold the wrist between your fingers and thumb, laying your thumb across the inner wrist. Now rock forward as you squeeze down the arm from wrist to elbow. Then rock back again and repeat the draining once or twice.

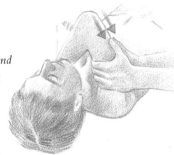

2 Draining the Upper Arm

Lift your partner's arm and let it bend at the elbow with the hand hanging down on the other side of the neck, so that the upper arm rises vertically. Grasp it near the elbow between both hands and pull down toward the shoulder joint, squeezing firmly. Repeat a couple of times.

Stretching

These "passive exercises" on the shoulder joint stretch and tone the connective tissues – the ligaments and tendons that attach the bones of the joint. They also stimulate the production of synovial fluid (the lubricant of the joints), and extend the joint's range of movement. As with any other "passive exercise", it is you that does the work here; your partner should surrender to the movement.

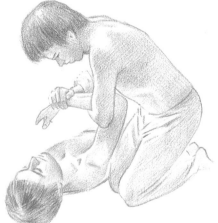

3 Lifting the Shoulder

Kneeling at your partner's shoulder, link one arm under the elbow joint (your left arm under their right and vice versa), making sure that the crooks of your arms are together. Take hold of your own opposite forearm near the elbow, and with your free hand anchor your partner's wrist. Now use your body to lift the arm, stretching the receiver's shoulder up off the floor. Bring it down gently. Repeat if you wish.

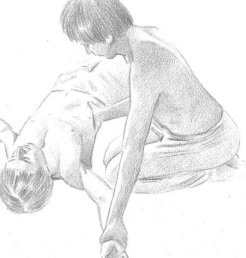

4 Stretching the Arm over the Head

Take hold of your partner's wrist and lift the arm above the head. Now pull gently on the wrist to give a final stretch to the arm while running your other hand firmly down the side of the ribcage from the armpit to stretch all the way along the arm and side.

Shoulder Joint and Arm

Having stretched the arm and shoulder joint, you now place the arm back by your partner's side and work around the shoulder girdle and down the arm. You begin with a stroke that squeezes from the centre of the upper chest and back out to the shoulder joint, then continue with some medium-depth work down the whole arm to the elbow and wrist. At the shoulder you are working on a ball and socket joint which has a wide range of movement, enabling the arm to swing round in a broad circle. The elbow is a hinge joint, which allows only an up-and-down movement. The bones of the forearm, however, can rotate over one another, and it is this that gives us the freedom to turn the palms of our hands up or down.

5 Squeezing the Shoulder Joint

A *Place one hand on the middle of your partner's upper chest, below the collarbone, the other under the upper back, just below the neck. Sandwiching the body between your hands, draw them slowly toward the shoulder joint, leading with the heels of your hands. Repeat this a few times.*

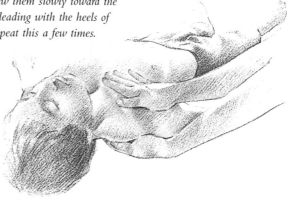

B *The final time that both hands reach the joint, curve them around the top of the arm and work deeply around the joint. Seek out the inner structures of bones and joint with your fingers.*

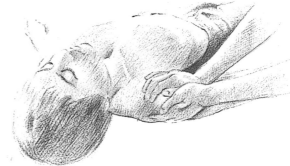

6 Kneading the Arm

Massage down the arm, kneading and wringing the whole limb until you reach the wrist. Give some attention to the elbow, exploring around the joint with your thumb and fingertips.

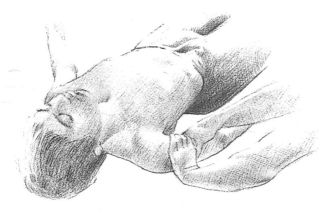

Wrist and Hand

A hand massage is especially relaxing – both because our hands are so accustomed to being touched and because, like the feet, the hands have reflex connections with the whole of the rest of the body (see p. 148). The area in the motor and sensory parts of the brain that is concerned with the hands is disproportionately large, indicating their unique sensitivity and functional importance. In fact, with their opposable thumbs, the hands are one of the main features that distinguish us from other animals. Pay special attention to the joints, for it is these that give the hands their great mobility.

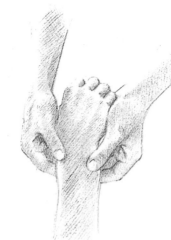

7 Working the Wrist

Lift your partner's forearm, resting the arm on the elbow. Now use your thumbs to work in small circles over the whole wrist area, holding the wrist between your thumbs and fingers.

8 Opening the Palm

Grasp the hand with your fingers on the palm and the heels of your hands on the back. Now squeeze and stretch the hand open by drawing your fingers away from one another while pressing the heels of your hands down. Repeat once or twice.
Note: *For the sake of clarity, this illustration is shown from below.*

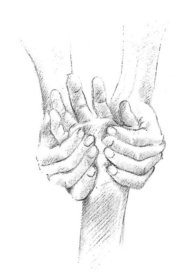

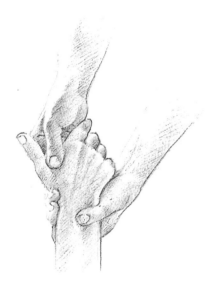

9 Cleaning between the Bones

Hold your partner's wrist to support the hand. Now use the thumb and index finger of your free hand to work along each of the grooves between the bones of the hand, from the wrist to the webs between the fingers.

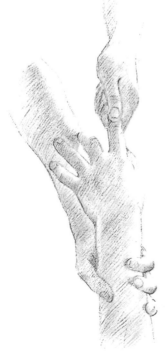

10 Wringing off the Fingers

Enclose the thumb and each of the fingers in turn in your hand and gently pull them, stretch them and twist them as you slide your hand down and off the tip. Now move over to the other side of your partner.

Repeat oiling and strokes 1–10 on the other arm.

Front of Torso

We face the world with the front of the body, exposing the belly, our most unprotected part. The front of the torso is linked to the way we feel and the way we relate. The torso consists of two main areas – the hard protective cage of the chest, which houses the heart, lungs and other organs, and the soft unprotected muscle wall of the belly, containing our guts – our deepest feelings. When massaging the front of the torso, be aware that this is an area of vulnerability. Before beginning, take a moment or two to study your partner's breathing pattern and observe which parts of the torso move with the breath, as you will be coordinating some of your strokes with the breathing. Our breathing pattern is intimately linked with our vitality and our emotional health. If your partner is trusting, having this area massaged can be a profound experience for both giver and receiver, establishing a deep contact between the two of you.

Oiling

For the oiling and long stroke on the front of the torso, you move to your partner's head. Always go gently over the solar plexus and belly, until you have a sense of how trusting your partner is. Some people are ticklish on their ribs and bellies. If your partner is one of them, avoid tight, small strokes and concentrate on slow, broad, firm ones.

Note: If using towels, bare the front of the torso, as shown on page 39.

Long Stroke

Rest your hands gently on the middle of the upper chest. Then rock forward from your hips, letting your hands slowly glide down the centre of the torso, allowing them to mould to the forms. Take care to avoid the breasts. Just below the navel, let your hands divide and curve out to the sides. Then rock back, pulling your hands back up the body along the sides. Repeat until the torso is oiled.

Broad Circling

Start as above, but when your hands divide on the abdomen, let them describe large overlapping circles as you travel smoothly up the sides.

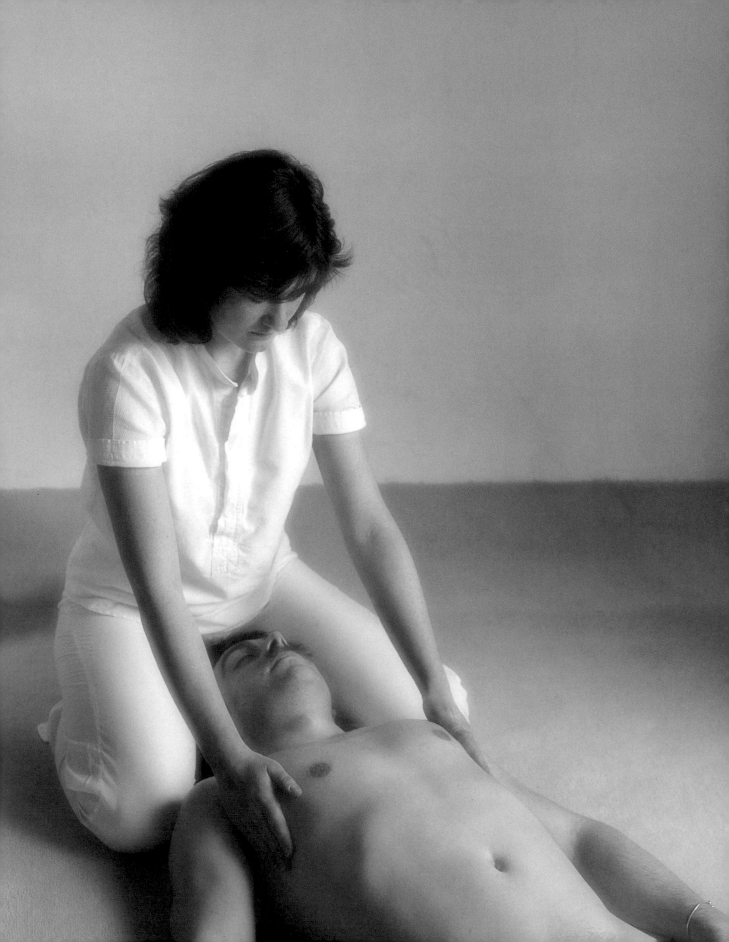

Ribcage and Chest

As well as protecting the vital organs in the upper chest, the ribcage plays an important part in the breathing process. We tend to think of the ribcage as fixed and static. But in fact, when we breathe in correctly, the ribs rise up, pushing the breastbone forward, and thus opening up the chest cavity, causing air to be drawn into the lungs. The muscles used in breathing are the large diaphragm muscle that crosses the body horizontally just below the ribcage, and those connecting the ribs themselves. To allow proper breathing, the diaphragm must be relaxed and the ribcage flexible. Massaging this area loosens the muscles and increases the mobility of the ribs. In this way it helps your partner to breathe more deeply.

1 Working between the Ribs

Positioned at your partner's head, place the first two fingers of both hands at the centre of the upper chest, in the grooves on either side of the topmost rib. Pressing firmly, draw your fingers out to the sides and off the body. Repeat, moving down to the grooves on either side of the rib below. Continue right down the ribcage in this way, as if tracing the rungs of a ladder. When you reach the bottom of the breastbone, you will find that the ribs no longer start at the centre and you must curve your hands round to work along them, as shown below right. Avoid working on the ribs that lie directly under the breasts. When you reach the breasts, press along the grooves for a short distance only, then move down to the next rib; don't press into the soft tissue of the breasts themselves. Continue the full stroke, once past the line of the breasts.

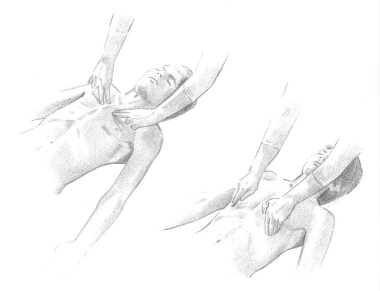

2 Pulling up the Sides

Leaning over your partner, use alternate strokes to pull up one side of the ribcage from the waist to the armpit. Work around, not directly across, the breasts.

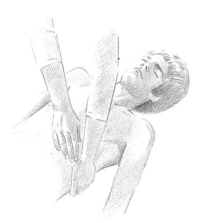

3 Kneading the Pectorals

Still working on the same side of the body, thoroughly knead the pectoral muscle — the muscle that forms the pit of the arm and supports the breast. Then slide your hands across the body and repeat the pulling-up and kneading strokes on the opposite side.

Repeat 2 and 3 on the other side.

The Abdomen

To work on the abdomen you move round to one side of your partner, level with the belly. The abdomen is highly sensitive, so let your hands come down gently initially and pause for a moment before you start. You begin by moving your hands in clockwise circles around the belly. It is important that you travel in a clockwise direction, for this echoes the direction of the large intestine. After rotating your hands over the belly in a broad circle, you gradually increase the depth of your pressure, using smaller circles. You end your massage on the front of the torso by working with the rhythm of your partner's breath. While your partner breathes slowly and deeply you glide your hands over the torso in a long circulatory stroke – up from the belly to the chest on an inhalation and down the sides on an exhalation. It is up to you to follow your partner's breath with your hands – not vice versa.

4 Broad Circling the Belly

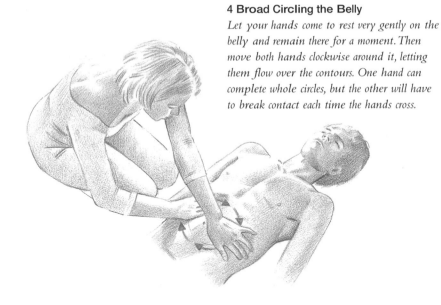

Let your hands come to rest very gently on the belly and remain there for a moment. Then move both hands clockwise around it, letting them flow over the contours. One hand can complete whole circles, but the other will have to break contact each time the hands cross.

5 Spiralling around the Belly

Still moving in a clockwise direction, divide your broad circles up into smaller ones, letting your hands spiral round as they travel over the belly.

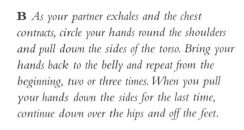

B *As your partner exhales and the chest contracts, circle your hands round the shoulders and pull down the sides of the torso. Bring your hands back to the belly and repeat from the beginning, two or three times. When you pull your hands down the sides for the last time, continue down over the hips and off the feet.*

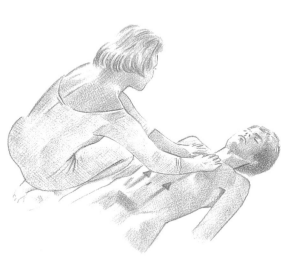

6 Long Stroke, using Breathing

A *Ask your partner to breathe slowly and deeply. Facing the head, rest your hands on the belly, fingers pointing up the body. As your partner inhales and the chest rises, slide your hands up the centre of the torso.*

Front of Legs

In Western society today, many of us have lost touch with our bodies, with the earth on which we stand. Too much of our time and energy is spent some way off the ground, living in our heads. A whole body massage ends on the feet, so that you bring the receiver's awareness right down to the toes and he or she leaves the massage session feeling "grounded". The sequence you follow is similar to the one you used on the backs of the legs. But here the terrain is a little different – as well as the soft muscle area of the thigh, you are working on the bony areas of the shin, and on the knee. Knees that are continually braced or pulled back indicate a somewhat insecure personality that is striving to maintain a hold on life and stand its ground. Massage can help release the energy blocked in the legs, allowing the person to move more freely through life.

Long Stroke on One Leg
Rest your hands on the ankle, fingers pointing up the leg, then let them glide slowly up, as you rock your body forward. When you near the top, curve your inner hand down the inside thigh while your other hand circles around the hip joint. Then rock backward, gliding both hands lightly down the sides of the leg and off the feet. Repeat until leg is oiled.

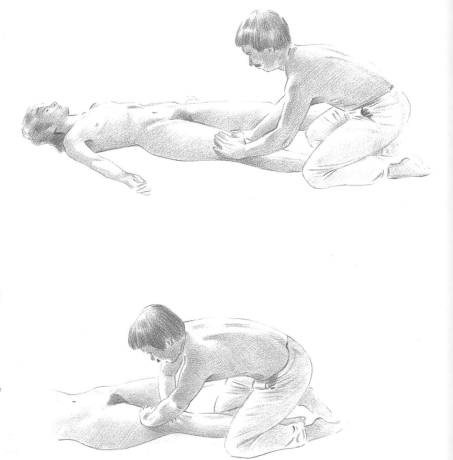

Oiling
Move down the receiver's body and position yourself between the feet. After applying oil to your hands you begin by oiling both legs. Rest your hands on your partner's ankles, then slide them all the way up the fronts of the legs to the top, around the hip joint and back down to the feet again. Repeat this stroke several times, then choose which leg you will work on first and position yourself on either side of the foot. Now you use both hands to spread the oil and warm the leg – either with your fingers pointing up the leg, as above, or with your hands cupped across it, as shown right. Take care to respect your partner's privacy, when working on the inner thigh.
Note: If using towels, uncover and oil one leg at a time (see p. 39).

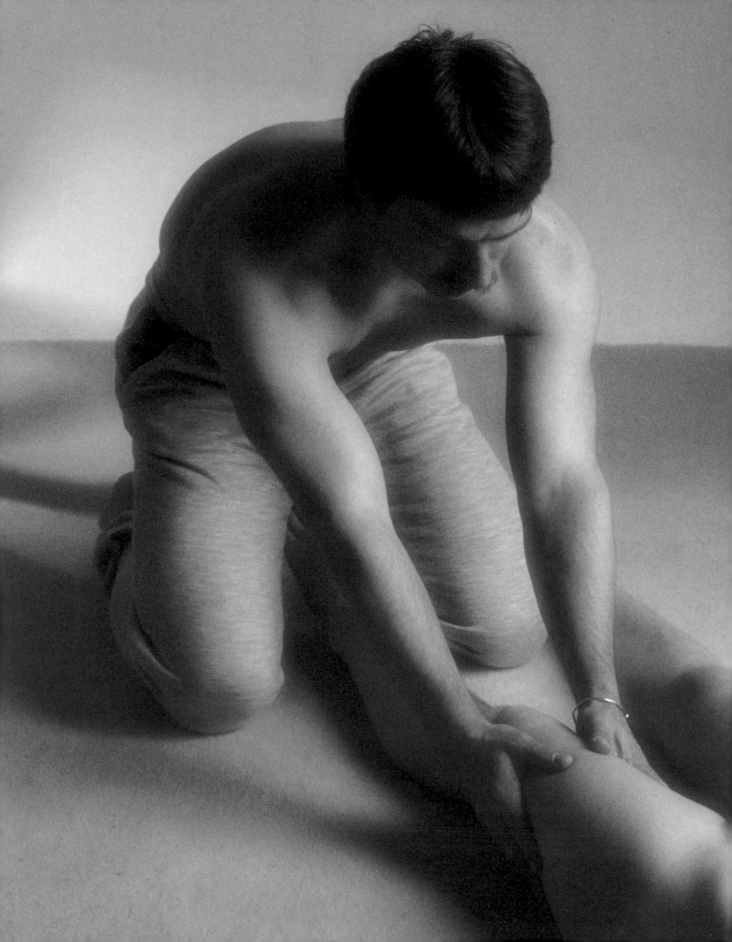

Stretching the Leg

When receiving a massage, it feels unexpectedly good to have your limbs passively exercised – like having someone do yoga for you, without you having to make any effort. In stretching the leg you are exercising three joints – the ball and socket hip joint and the hinge joints of knee and ankle. As the giver, you will find it more effective and less tiring if you pull with your whole body, not just your arms. And make sure that your grip on the foot is comfortable to your partner.

1 Stretching the Leg

Cup one hand around your partner's heel, the other across the top of the foot. Lean back until your arms are taut, like ropes. Now raise the foot a few centimetres (inches) and lean back from your pelvis, shaking the leg slightly as you pull. Release slowly then repeat once.

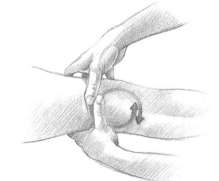

2 Draining the Lower Leg

Use the "V" between your thumbs and fingers to press firmly along the muscles on either side of the shinbone. Move your hands alternately, letting one follow the other rhythmically up from ankle to knee. Repeat several times.

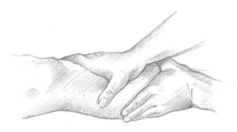

Working up the Front of the Leg

This sequence basically consists of draining strokes to aid the circulation, interspersed with some more precise work around the kneecap. On the lower leg, you must be sure to work on the muscles on either side of the shinbone. Direct pressure on the shinbone can be painful for the receiver. On the thigh, you use broad, fairly deep strokes to push upward, assisting the venous and lymphatic flow. If your partner has long legs, you may find it impossible to reach the thigh unless you move to the side.

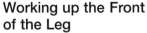

3 Circling the Kneecap *(left)*

Overlap your thumbs just above the kneecap, anchoring your fingers on the sides of the knee. Simultaneously draw your thumbs away from each other to circle around the bone from opposite directions, letting them cross above and below the kneecap. Circle several times.

4 Draining the Thigh *(right)*

Use both hands to push alternately up the thigh from the knee to the top of the leg. Let your thumbs circle up and outward as you move gradually up the leg. Repeat several times.

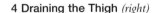

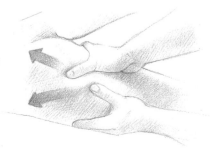

The Hip Joint and down the Leg

Linking the top of the leg to the pelvis, the hip joint is a large ball and socket joint with a wide range of movement. It is packed in firmly by the surrounding muscles, and may be hard to find at first. Press in under the rim of the pelvis to locate the bony protuberance at the top of the thigh bone (see p. 181). If you delve deeper round this bone, you will be working on the connections of the hip joint. Having pressed around the joint thoroughly, you now work down the leg, using broad strokes on the thigh, more precise finger strokes around the kneecap, and then finish by squeezing down the shin muscles to the ankle. As you work down the leg, you will need to move. When working on a massage table it is easy to move smoothly; but if working on the floor you will probably have to break contact gently, change position, then continue.

5 Working around the Hip Joint

Facing your partner's hip, place both your thumbs on the side of the buttocks, 5–7.5 cm (2–3 in) below the rim of the pelvis. Now knead around the joint, pushing in deeply with alternate thumbs. Use the rest of your hands to "anchor" you.

6 Working down the Leg

Gather and squeeze large bunches of flesh down the thigh, then wring or pull along it. Work around the knee with your fingers, then continue down the lower leg, squeezing alongside the shinbone to the ankle joint.

The Front of the Foot

You round off a massage session with some final attention to the feet, moving down to sit or stand facing the foot you are working on. As you have already massaged them thoroughly while the receiver was lying on their back, these strokes are simply intended to "ground" your partner, bringing the energy right down. After first opening and stretching the foot, you enclose it in both hands and pull them soothingly off the toes. Then you position yourself on either side of the receiver's other foot to work on the other leg.

7 Opening the Foot

Clasp the foot with your fingers under the sole and your thumbs alongside one another on the top. Squeezing the foot firmly, draw the lengths of your thumbs away from each other, opening the foot and stretching the bones apart.

8 Stroking the Foot

Sandwich the foot between your hands, fingers pointing up the leg. Draw them slowly toward you and slide gently off the toes. Repeat this finishing stroke a few times.

Repeat 1–8 on the other leg.

Connecting

Having worked on each part of the body in turn, you now need to "connect" the various parts and give your partner a sense of wholeness. There are two ways of connecting the body – by long strokes which flow over the entire body, from one end to the other; or by simply resting your two hands on different parts of the body for a few moments. You may also use these connecting strokes as a bridge between working on one part of the body and the next. The "held" stroke can connect any parts of the body you choose – for example, the forehead and belly, as shown opposite, or the belly or base of the spine and the feet. After the connecting strokes, cover your partner with a warmed towel and leave him or her to rest for a while. If you have been working with towels, make sure your partner is fully covered and then do light connecting strokes over the towels to finish.

Long Connecting Strokes

For these final connecting strokes, you should position yourself by your partner's side, at hip level, so that you can reach both ends of the body at once. You can either do just one of the strokes given below and right, or all three if you wish. But whichever stroke you end with, let your fingers rest for a moment before breaking contact and then gently release both hands together.

Belly to Leg and Arm

Rest both hands on your partner's belly, then slowly (moving both hands simultaneously) glide one hand down one leg and off the foot and the other up to the opposite shoulder, down the arm, and off the hand. Bring the hands back to the belly and repeat the stroke along the other leg and arm.

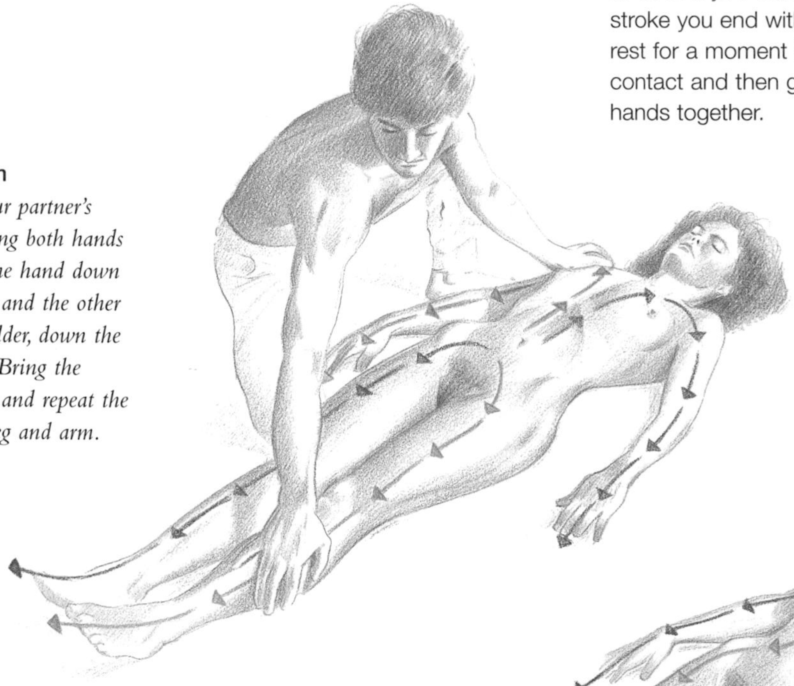

Head to Hands and Feet

Rest your fingertips on the forehead, then move lightly up over the top of the head, down the back of the neck, down the arms and off the fingertips. Repeat, but at the base of the neck, come round to the front and down the torso. At the navel, separate your hands and come down the legs and off the toes.

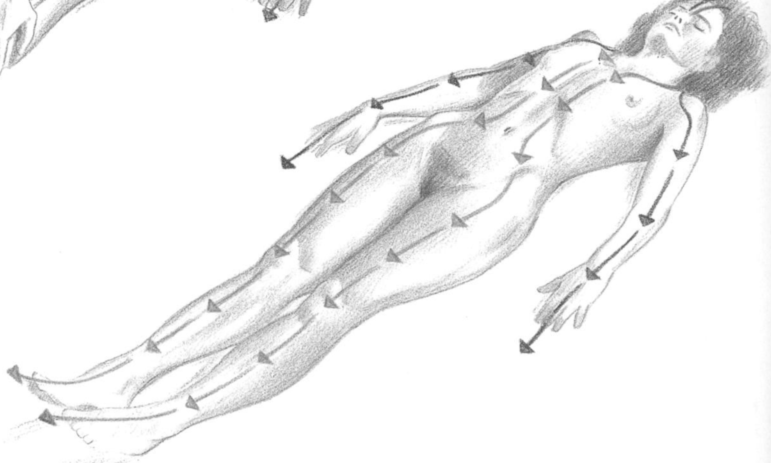

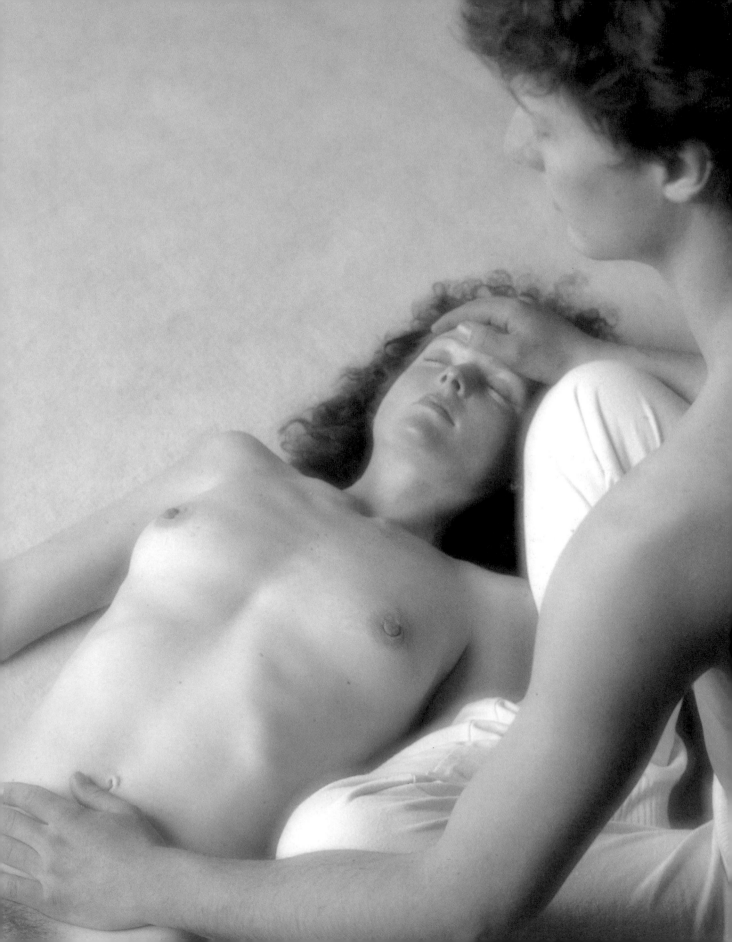

Massage Checklist

This chart is intended to remind you, both visually and verbally, of the strokes in the massage sequence, and of the stages at which you change your own or your partner's position. The complete sequence will take you about an hour to an hour and a half, but there is no need always to stick to it rigidly. Sometimes, for instance, you may find that you want to spend longer on an area that is particularly tense or one that feels especially good to the receiver. On other occasions, you may not have enough time for a long massage and will want to do a shorter version, choosing just a few parts to work on thoroughly – say, the back, arms and hands, and feet. Consult your partner as to what he or she would prefer. But be sure to give at least some long strokes to the parts that you don't massage – otherwise your partner will feel disconnected.

Note: In these illustrations, the arrow indicates the position of the giver and the shaded area represents the part of the body worked on.

Back of Body
The Back (pp. 40–5)

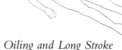

Oiling and Long Stroke

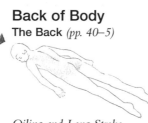

1 *Kneading the Shoulder*
2 *Thumb-rolling at Base of Neck*
3 *Thumbing beside the Spine*

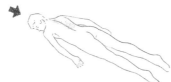

4 *Working under the Rim of the Blade*
5 *Pressing the Flat of the Blade*
6 *Squeezing the Spine of the Blade*
7 *Kneading the Neck*

Repeat 1–7 on the other side

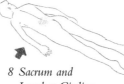

8 *Sacrum and Lumbar Circling*

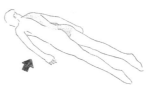

9 *Kneading the Buttocks*
10 *Plucking the Buttocks*
11 *Pulling up the Sides*

Repeat 9–11 on the other side

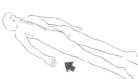

12 *"Rocking Horse"*
13 *Friction along the Spine*
14 *Forearm Pressure*

Back of Legs (pp. 46–51)

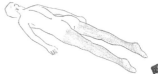

Oiling and Long Stroke on Both Legs

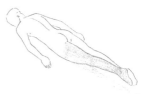

Oiling and Long Stroke on One leg
1 *Leg Lifting*
2 *Draining with Thumbs*
3 *Draining with Heels of Hands*

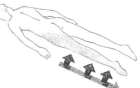

4 *Kneading the Leg*
5 *Wringing along the Leg*

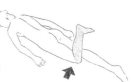

6 *Working around the Ankle*
7 *Rotating the Ankle*
8 *Pushing the Foot Down and Up*
9 *Cleaning between the Tendons*
10 *Thumbing the Sole*
11 *Stretching the Toes*
12 *Wringing the Toes*

Repeat oiling and strokes 1–12 on the other leg

Front of Body

Shoulders, Neck, and Scalp *(pp. 52–7)*

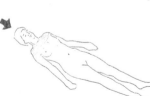

Oiling and Long Stroke

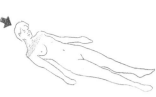

1 *Stretching the Neck*
2 *Stretching the Neck Up and Down*
3 *Stretching the Neck from Side to Side*

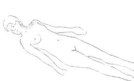

4 *Shoulder, Front, and Back Sequence*

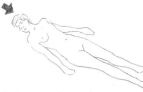

5 *Rotating the Scalp*
6 *"Shampooing"*
7 *"Pulling off" the Hair*

Repeat 4–7 on the other side

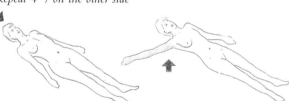

8 *Spinal Stretch*

The Face *(pp. 58–62)*

1 Forehead
2 Eyebrows
3 Eyes
4 Nose
5 Cheeks
6 Chin
7 Jawbone
8 Chewing Muscles
9 Cheek to Ear Stroke
10 Connecting the Face and the Head

Arms and Hands *(pp. 63–7)*

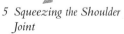

Oiling and Long Stroke

1 *Draining the Forearm*

2 *Draining the Upper Arm*
3 *Lifting the Shoulder*

4 *Stretching the Arm over the Head*

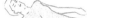
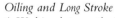
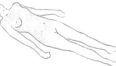

5 *Squeezing the Shoulder Joint*
6 *Kneading the Arm*
7 *Working the Wrist*
8 *Opening the Palm*
9 *Cleaning between the Bones*
10 *Wringing off the Fingers*

Repeat oiling and strokes 1–10 on the other arm

Front of Torso *(pp. 68–71)*

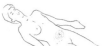

Oiling and Long Stroke
1 *Working between the Ribs*
2 *Pulling up the Sides*
3 *Kneading the Pectorals*

Repeat 2 and 3 on the other side

4 *Broad Circling the Belly*
5 *Spiralling around the Belly*

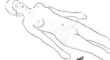

6 *Long Stroke, using Breathing*

Front of Legs *(pp. 72–5)*

Oiling and Long Stroke on Both Legs

Oiling and Long Stroke on One Leg
1 *Stretching the Leg*
2 *Draining the Lower Leg*
3 *Circling the Kneecap*
4 *Draining the Thigh*

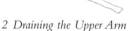

5 *Working around the Hip Joint*
6 *Working down the Leg*
7 *Opening the Foot*
8 *Stroking the Foot*

Repeat 1–8 on the other leg

Connecting *(pp. 76–7)*

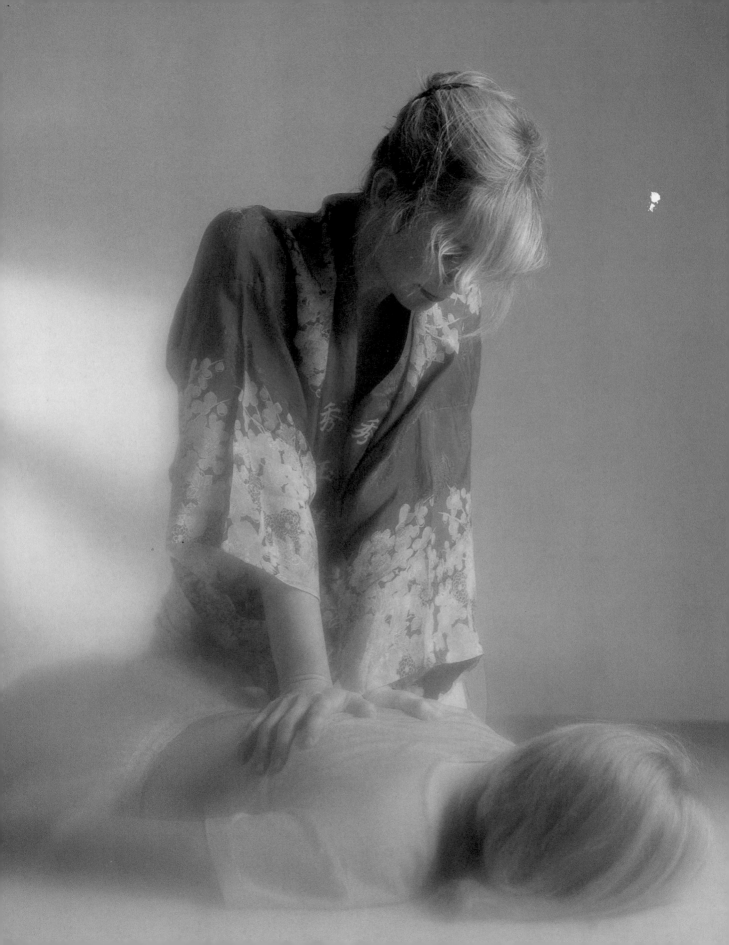

Shiatsu

Shiatsu comes from Japan. It is a form of physical therapy that involves pressure on the acupuncture points in order to balance the body's energy and promote good health. Although its name means simply "finger pressure", shiatsu is also applied with other parts of the hand, as well as with the elbows and knees.

The art was given its name around the turn of the century, although its origins are ancient. It is a unique combination of classical Oriental medical theory, whose history stretches back to the beginnings of acupuncture 4000 years ago, and a rich living tradition of folk medicine.

Shiatsu is the generic name for a wide variety of techniques, but all practitioners are linked by a common principle, the belief in a vital force known as *ki* which flows in connected channels or "meridians" throughout the body. Each meridian is linked to an organ or psycho-physical function, and its *ki* can be contacted at certain points along its path – these are the acupuncture points known in Japanese as *tsubos*. In health, a balanced condition prevails, and the *ki* flows smoothly along the meridians, like fuel through a pipeline, supplying and maintaining all parts of the body. But when the body has been weakened by an immoderate lifestyle (see p. 86), emotional stress or injury, the *ki* no longer flows smoothly, becoming deficient in some areas and excessive in others and a state of disease exists.

Most of us fall into the category of "half-healthy" people – in other words, our condition is not completely balanced. We may be liable to colds or stomach upsets, or get moody and depressed. For such "half-healthy" people, or as a preventive against sickness, shiatsu is the ideal home remedy since it simply rebalances the *ki* so that the body can heal itself.

When beginning shiatsu it is important to bear in mind that you are aiming to treat not only your partner's symptoms, but also their cause. To treat only the head for a headache is to ignore not only the whole supporting system of interconnecting meridians which makes shiatsu so effective, but also one of the fundamental principles of Oriental medicine – that body and mind are an indivisible, organic whole. To diagnose the exact cause of a person's symptoms requires both a thorough grasp of Oriental medical theory and an understanding of that person's emotional and psychological condition. Until such skills have been acquired, it is safer and more effective to treat the whole body.

As mentioned above, all diseases are caused by an excess or deficiency of *ki*. With practice you will learn to sense by touch the areas which show an excess of *ki*, called *jitsu*, and those where *ki* is deficient, which are called *kyo* (see p. 85). Usually the *jitsu*, or painful area, is the symptom and the *kyo* area the cause, so you will treat partners most effectively if you concentrate on *kyo* areas in your shiatsu. The "*kyo-jitsu*" method of treatment was advocated by the late Master Shizuto Masunaga as an alternative to the established school, which recommended formulae, or combinations of *tsubos*, for the treatment of specific problems.

Shiatsu is easy to learn. No special equipment is required and no oil is used. All you need is a warm airy room, loose comfortable clothing for both giver and receiver, and a carpeted floor to work on. You can safely give shiatsu anywhere, and as often as once a day. A little background knowledge, the time to give a full body treatment, attention and sensitivity toward your partner – this is all you need to begin to feel your way toward a real understanding of shiatsu.

Ki

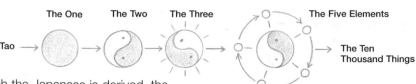

The One   The Two   The Three   The Five Elements

Tao   The Ten
Thousand Things

In Chinese cosmology, from which the Japanese is derived, the source of all things is the *tao*, the law of the universe. From the *tao* derives the one, or existence. Two forces polarize from this, the *yin* and the *yang*, which are both opposite and complementary. It is the play between the *yin* and the *yang*, the ebb and the flow between the two principles, which creates *ki* energy (or *chi*, as the Chinese call it), and thus the two become the three. *Ki* is the "immaterial breath" of which Lao Tzu writes in the *Tao Te Ching* (see right). It exists in many forms, from the purest, such as light, to the grossest, such as granite, for even inert material is made of *ki* in its densest form, just as all matter is made of particles of energy. How do the "three beget the ten thousand things"? According to ancient philosophy, *ki* manifests itself as five different aspects of energy, known as the Five Elements – Fire, Earth, Metal, Water, and Wood. Each element has its own particular quality or "flavour", and imparts it to some aspect of creation, to one of the "ten thousand things". Plant life, for example, belongs mainly to the Wood element, rocks and minerals to the Metal element. Human beings are a blend of all five elements. Everything in nature, each of the ten thousand things, is composed of a particular blend of *yin* and *yang*, together with a particular combination of the five elements, which is unique, which forms the "true *ki*" of that object or being.

"The tao begets the one,
The one begets the two
The two beget the three and
The three beget the ten thousand things.
All things are backed by the shade,
Faced by the light
And harmonized by the immaterial breath."

           Lao Tzu: Tao Te Ching

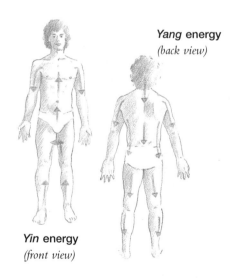

Yang energy
(back view)

Yin energy
(front view)

Yin and Yang Meridians

The yin *and* yang *meridians of the body are said to have been formed when we were still running on all fours. Earth is* yin *in relation to heaven. So the* yin *meridians run up the front and inside body surfaces, which would have been closest to the earth. Heaven is* yang *in relation to earth, so the* yang *meridians run down the back and outside surfaces which would have been exposed to sunlight.*

Yin and Yang

Yin and *yang* are the two opposite yet complementary aspects of existence – the shade and the light. *Yin* corresponds to that which is dark, cool, moist, soft, receptive, feminine, and sinking; *yang* to that which is light, hot, dry, hard, active, masculine, and rising. *Yin* and *yang* are only relative conditions, however, not absolutes, so one thing can be *yin* to another and *yang* in relation to a third. For example, a candle is *yang* compared with an icecube but *yin* compared with the sun. In Oriental medicine, the nourishing, cooling, moistening, relaxing functions are *yin*, the active, heat-producing energetic aspects of functioning *yang*. The substance of the organs is mostly *yin*, the energy that supplies them is *yang*. Where there is too much *yin*, there is a tendency to coldness, dampness and condensation into substance (for example the formation of tumours). With too much *yang* there is overactivity and heat. When *yin* is deficient, even though the *yang* energy may be normal, there will be *yang*-type symptoms, such as nervous excitability, insomnia, a dry mouth, and so on. When *yang* is deficient, there will be tiredness, chilliness and poor circulation. The beauty of shiatsu is that, when given with sensitivity to your partner's individual needs, it will automatically balance your partner's energy.

The Five Elements

The Five Elements are the different qualities of *ki* energy, the five different modes in which it manifests itself in the universe. The elements also manifest themselves in humans, linking us with the rest of the environment, with the cycle of the seasons and the hours. The way we respond, physically and emotionally, to external influences and to the forces of nature depends on the balance of the elements within us. Fire is the element of heat, summer, enthusiasm, and warmth in human relationships. Earth is the element of harvest time, abundance, nourishment, fertility, and the mother–child relationship. Metal includes the Western idea of the air element, but it is more. It is the force of gravity, the minerals within the earth, the patterns of the heavenly bodies, the powers of electrical conductivity and magnetism. In man it is grief and the yearning to transcend it. Water is the source of life, the capacity to flow, infinitely yielding yet infinitely powerful, ever-changing and often dangerous. It is the most *yin* of the elements. In human psychology, Water governs the balance between fear and the desire to dominate. Wood is the most human of the elements. It is the element of spring, and the creative urge to achieve, which turns to anger when frustrated. In man it is the capacity to look forward, plan and make decisions.

Each element governs a meridian or organ function in the human body (as shown above right) and also an aspect of the personality or emotions, so that any disturbance of the elements will affect the mind and body in specific ways. The value of an understanding of the elements to a doctor of Oriental medicine is that the network of element associations provides clues on which he can base a diagnosis.

Each element is associated with a colour, a taste, a season, a smell, an emotion, and a sound (see above). So

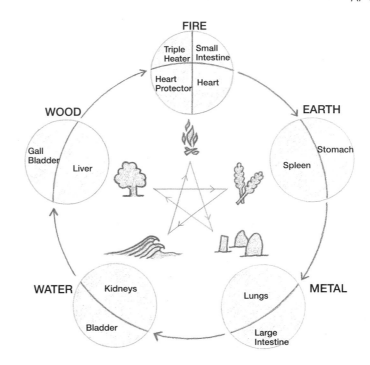

The Associations and Meridians of the Five Elements and their Cycles

Each element is related to all four others via the "creative cycle" (outer arrows) and the "control cycle" (inner arrows). In the creative cycle each element passes energy on to the next. The control cycle counterbalances it, so that the elements are held in check.

Elements	Fire	Earth	Metal	Water	Wood
Colour	red	yellow	white	blue/black	green
Sound	laughing	singing	weeping	groaning	shouting
Odour	scorched	fragrant	rotten	putrid	rancid
Emotion	joy	sympathy	grief	fear	anger
Season	summer	late summer	autumn	winter	spring
Taste	bitter	sweet	pungent	salty	sour

the doctor will not only be interested in the patient's symptoms, he will also have learned to perceive subtle hues of colour on the face, to distinguish inflections in the voice, and to make accurate judgements on the patient's emotional state. He can then confirm his diagnosis by questioning. What kind of taste does the patient crave? What weather makes the condition worse? In this way he sees beyond the symptoms to the cause, which lies in one of the elements. If the diagnosis points to the Water element, the doctor will know he must treat the kidneys and bladder; the same symptoms in another patient may stem from the Earth element, so the doctor will treat the spleen and stomach. A Western doctor would most likely label both patients "arthritic" and prescribe anti-inflammatory drugs.

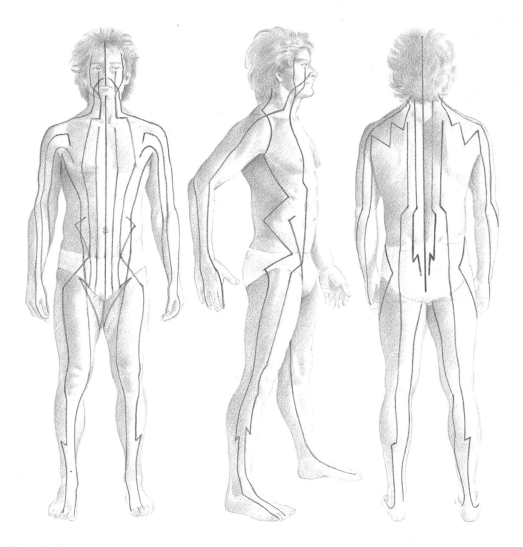

The Meridians

The meridians are channels along which *ki* flows through the body. The best known are the twelve meridians of acupuncture. The Five Elements have a pair of meridians each, one *yin* and one *yang*, except for Fire, which has two pairs. All twelve meridians are bilateral, making twenty-four in all. The paired meridians run close to each other, and their functions are complementary. Each meridian is associated with a particular organ or psycho-physical function, but in its effect it extends far beyond the activity of the organ as Western science understands it. For instance

the Liver Meridian is associated with the nails, the muscles and tendons, the reproductive system, the emotion of anger, the eyes, the ability to plan, and so on. You don't need a detailed understanding of the meridian associations at the beginning; but you should understand that if the Liver Meridian, say, is painful or tense, it is not necessarily the liver *organ* that is in trouble, but the Liver energy. Two "extra" meridians are usually included with the twelve organ meridians; the Governing Vessel, which is a kind of reservoir of *yang* energy, and the Conception Vessel, its *yin* counterpart.

When you press a point on a meridian, you are not only stimulating the local nerves and tissues, but influencing the flow of *ki* throughout that meridian and thence through others. If an area is too painful to touch, you can help by working on areas further along the meridians which cross the painful area. With the bilateral meridians, you can also affect the flow of *ki* to a painful area by working on the same place on the opposite side. Points near the ends of a meridian are often the most powerful in removing blocks or relieving pain along the course of that meridian.

The *Tsubos*

The acupuncture points or *tsubos* are places on the meridian where *ki* can be most easily reached and manipulated. These points have been proved to have a lower electrical resistance than the surrounding areas. The *tsubos* act a little like amplifiers, passing the *ki* from one point to another. Many of the *tsubos* are what the West calls "trigger points" which stimulate the muscle to contract or relax. But the *tsubos* have much subtler effects according to the laws of *ki*. Some connect with other meridians, some influence the balance of the elements, others may calm the mind or reduce fever. In this book we lay more emphasis on the meridians than on the *tsubos*. If you learn the whereabouts of the meridians, you will become familiar with the "feel" of the pathways of *ki* within the body, and will develop an instinctive knowledge of where the *tsubos* are. And if the point you intuitively press does not appear in the acupuncture charts, it is nonetheless valid if your partner feels benefit from it.

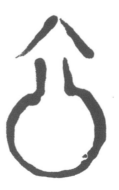

The Symbol for *Tsubo*
The ancient Chinese character for "tsubo" represents a jar with a narrow neck and a cover. The tsubo *is like the neck of the jar — under the covering lies the "way in" to the storehouse of* ki.

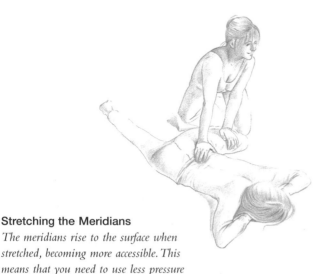

Stretching the Meridians
The meridians rise to the surface when stretched, becoming more accessible. This means that you need to use less pressure when giving shiatsu to a stretched limb.

Kyo and *Jitsu*

In a meridian which is out of balance, *ki* can be either deficient *(kyo)* or in excess *(jitsu)* and sometimes, where the *ki* flow is obstructed, it can be both at once – in excess above the obstruction and deficient below it. *Kyo* areas often look and feel slightly hollow and are usually yielding to the touch. When you press a *kyo* meridian it generally feels good to your partner, as you are supplying *ki* energy to a deficiency. *Jitsu* areas are much easier to find, as they are usually hard or tense. They may be spontaneously painful, or they may only feel painful when pressed. The pain is generally sharp, whereas *kyo* pain is usually dull and gives relief when you press it – a "good hurt". Shiatsu treatment is far more pleasant and effective when you concentrate on the *kyo* areas. This technique, known as "tonification", uses slow and gradual pressure to impart energy to the deficiency. In principle, every excess symptom is caused by a deficiency, so that tonifying the *kyo* meridians will help the *jitsu* ones to relax.

The Oriental Way of Health

To give good shiatsu, you must have good quality *ki* yourself. According to ancient philosophy, your basic constitution is determined by your "prenatal *ki*", which is received at the moment of conception, and depends upon the age and health of your parents, although it is also affected by the circumstances of your birth. This prenatal *ki*, which is stored in the kidney area, can never be added to. It can only be depleted by an unwise lifestyle or, at best, conserved by a wise one. There is only one way of preserving this precious reservoir, and that is *moderation*. Any obvious abuse of the body, such as drug-taking, consistent late nights, or long-term overwork, depletes it. In women it is also depleted by childbearing and, in men, by sexual activity. "Postnatal *ki*", however, is a constant inflow of energy. It is the *ki* that we receive from earth, by eating, and from heaven, by breathing, and so particular attention should be paid to both of these.

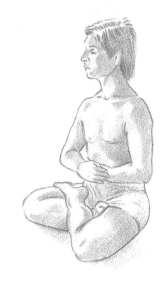

Diet

To practise shiatsu, you should have a balanced, healthy diet. The keyword is moderation. Keep a balance between the five tastes – sweet, salty, bitter, sour, and hot. You don't need to be macrobiotic or vegetarian, but meat and fish should be kept to a minimum and balanced by whole grains and vegetables. Raw food diets are fine for cleansing the system, but they are not a good long-term proposition. Living on salads will not supply you with enough *yang* energy, so no more than a third of your diet should be raw, except in very hot weather. Avoid ice cream and any food or drink straight from the fridge, as the cold impairs the ability of the Spleen and Stomach functions. And cut down on dairy products, particularly if you suffer from catarrh, chestiness or allergies.

Breathing

It is a good idea to do some breathing exercises each day – either yogic breathing or breathing into the abdomen or *hara*, as shown above. For this, sit cross-legged or Japanese-style, kneeling with your feet tucked under you. Place your left hand on your *hara* and your right hand over it. Inhale into the *hara* for 5 seconds. Hold your breath for 5 seconds, then exhale from the *hara* for 5 seconds. Repeat for up to 10 minutes, imagining your *hara* as a glowing sphere, with more *ki* accumulating there with each breath.

Stimulants and Drugs

Coffee, tea, alcohol and cigarettes are all drugs which help us to cope with the pressures of life, but all in different ways take their toll on the body. All are harmful to the Kidney energy, especially coffee, while alcohol often affects the Liver and cigarettes the Lungs. Obviously it would be best to cut them out altogether, but since your aim is moderation, don't attempt to give everything up all at once. Instead, retrain yourself to appreciate these substances in small quantities. You could cut coffee down to one cup in the morning to wake you up and reduce smoking to three cigarettes a day. Try to cultivate awareness of your body and its needs, rather than imposing strict regimes which can often lead to an overreaction in the opposite direction.

Exercise

Some form of exercise is a necessity, especially if you find yourself doing a lot of shiatsu, in which case you will need to keep fit. All exercise is beneficial, but if you want to increase your *ki*, you will need an Oriental system which works with "subtle energy". Hatha yoga is an excellent form of exercise which stretches all the meridians and regulates the breathing. T'ai chi is also designed to increase your *ki*, improve your breathing and make your body soft and flexible. Both these different kinds of *ki*-increasing exercise are really a form of self-shiatsu, and may ultimately be more enjoyable and beneficial than trying to press your own meridians.

Protecting Your Body

It is essential to remember to protect yourself against external conditions. The Chinese and Japanese recognize wind, cold, damp, and heat as disease-producing factors and protect themselves accordingly. It is particularly important to keep the neck and shoulders and the lumbar region warm, so make sure that your shirt doesn't leave a gap at the waist when you bend over, and wear a scarf when you go out on cold or windy days. And if you have trouble spots such as painful knees or ankles, keep them warm. Oriental medicine has long recognized that "half-healthy" people should not court trouble from the elements.

Emotional Factors

At the other end of the spectrum come the emotional or psychological factors which can affect your health. In the Oriental system, worry, grief, fear, anger, even too much joy are all possible causes of disease. But since fighting these distur-bances creates even more conflict, the Oriental way is to observe them with awareness and allow them to be. In this way they will naturally quieten and abate, just as a restless horse, let loose in a large meadow, will eventually become calm and begin to graze. Meditation is the time-honoured Eastern way of achieving this end. For the shiatsu practitioner, this is surely one of the hardest but most rewarding tasks – to understand and feel compassion for one's own troubles and anxiety in order to have more under-standing and compassion for those of other people.

Tools and Techniques

Shiatsu techniques could not be more different from those used in most Western forms of massage – there are no smooth flowing strokes, no kneading or friction. In fact, only two main techniques are used – pressure and stretching. And yet it is an immensely dynamic and varied form of massage. The variety comes from the different "tools" used for applying pressure (hands, elbows, knees and feet), from the durations and depths of pressure, and from the positions in which the receiver's limbs are placed. The key to good shiatsu technique is to be as natural and relaxed as possible in applying pressure. This means using your body weight in a controlled but effortless way, rather than consciously "pressing", and making sure that you always keep both hands in contact with the receiver's body.

Correct Shiatsu Technique

This is the right position for giving shiatsu. The knees are apart, providing a steady base; the arms are straight, providing firm support; and the pressure is coming not from the shoulders, which are relaxed, but from the forward movement of the hips. Both the giver's hands are relaxed.

Coming from the *Hara*

In correct shiatsu technique, pressure comes from the *hara* (the centre of energy in the lower belly, see p. 122), regardless of which "tool" you are using to apply the pressure. Pressure from the *hara* is controlled and considerate, because your energy is sensitive to that of your partner. The best way of learning this basic art is to use your body weight, allowing your partner to support you, as shown right, rather than "pressing" with effort. Your own body position is crucial. You should be relaxed and rock steady. In this way you can apply firm pressure without tiring.

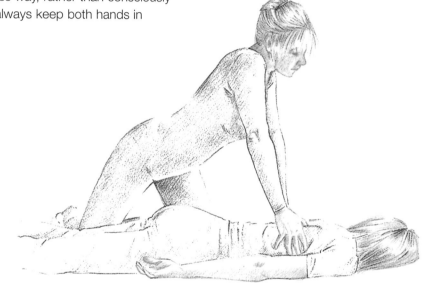

Incorrect Shiatsu Technique

This is the wrong way to give shiatsu. The knees are together, giving no stability; only one hand is applying deep pressure, so the reassurance that comes from two-handed contact is lacking; the arm is bent, involving more muscular effort; and the movement is obviously coming from the shoulder (which is tense), not from the hips. The giver's whole body is strained and will soon tire.

The Tools of Shiatsu

The thumbs are the classic shiatsu tools, since the *tsubos*, or pressure points, are often located in thumb-sized hollows. But using your thumbs throughout a shiatsu session would be tiring – and different tools provide variety for both giver and receiver. Try to save using your thumbs for occasions when you need to apply precise pressure on key points; use your hands, knees or elbows for pressing down the meridian lines.

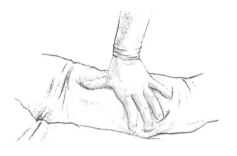

Thumbs
When using your thumbs in shiatsu, let the ball, not the tip, apply pressure, and allow the rest of the hand to remain in contact with the receiver's body – both to help support your weight and to reassure your partner.

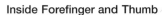

Inside Forefinger and Thumb
This is known as the "dragon's mouth" hold and is very useful for those with flexible hands. Pressure falls mainly on the lowest joint of the index finger.

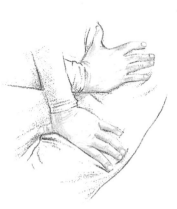

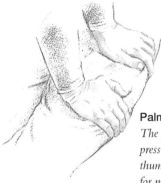

Palms
The palm of the hand provides good pressure, but is less specific than the thumbs. Use the heel of your hand for more precision, but keep the rest of your hand in relaxed contact.

Knees
Knee pressure should feel strong but not painful. Stay back on your haunches and bounce lightly and repeatedly. Don't kneel on your partner!

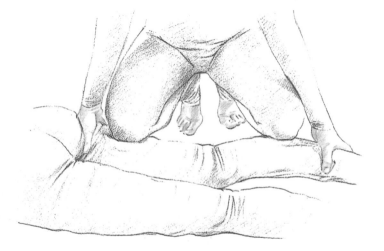

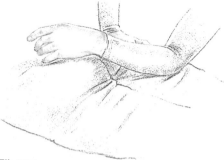

Elbows
When using your elbow to apply pressure, keep your knees apart and your centre of gravity low to give yourself more control. Make sure that your elbow is "open" – a sharp elbow is painful – and your hand and forearm are relaxed. A tense fist indicates that you are consciously "pressing".

Basic Shiatsu Sequence

You start the sequence with the receiver lying prone, arms by the sides. Working down the body, you first treat the back, then the hips, then the back of the legs and feet, before returning to the head end to give shiatsu to the back of the shoulders. Make sure that your partner turns his or her head frequently to avoid getting a stiff neck. On the front of the body, you systematically treat the front of the shoulders and neck, the head and the face, the arms and the hands and the *hara*, finishing on the front of the legs. People with lower back problems may prefer to keep their legs raised when lying on their backs, lowering them when you come to work on their legs.

Caution: *Avoid pressing directly on the veins, if your partner has varicose veins. And avoid shiatsu on the abdomen during pregnancy. In the later stages of pregnancy, avoid heavy pressure on the legs, and don't use the "Great Eliminator" (see p. 121).*

1 Back

You begin by stretching the back, to loosen it and to establish your own rhythm. Next you stimulate all the body functions by applying pressure down both sides of the spine with your palms, then your thumbs.

2 Hips

On the hips you press the points in the sacrum, then squeeze the sides of the buttocks, and use your elbow on the upper curve.

4 Back of Shoulders

Your shiatsu on the back of the body ends with the shoulders. You press along the top of each shoulder, then rotate the shoulderblades. Now you treat the area between the spine and shoulderblades and finish by loosening the shoulder muscles with your feet.

Your partner now turns over.

3 Back of Legs

Working on one leg at a time, you press down the centre with your palm, then your knees. After pressing the ankle points, you stretch the leg three ways, then crook it outward to press down the side. Next you walk on your partner's soles then treat each foot in turn.

5 Front of Shoulders

First you "open" the chest by leaning on the front of the shoulders, then press along the spaces between the ribs to relieve congestion in the chest and help to correct rounded shoulders. Resting your elbows on your knees for leverage, you work on the meridians on the back of the neck from below, then circle the sides of the neck to loosen the muscles. Stretching the neck completes this sequence.

6 Head and Face

Starting at the top of the head, you run your fingers through the hair and gently pull it. After massaging the ears, you work systematically down the points on the face – round the eyes, on the temples and jaw, near the nostrils and mouth – then back along the midline of the head.

7 Arms and Hands

One arm at a time, you first treat the inner surface, with the hand palm up, then the forearm, with the hand palm down. Now you pull the fingers and treat the important point between thumb and forefinger, ending by shaking the arm to loosen and relax it.

8 *Hara*

Using both hands you work clockwise round the lower hara *then press gently under both sides of the ribs and down the midline to the navel. Now relax the* hara *by rocking it.*

9 Front of Legs

Working down toward the feet each time, you press down the inside of the leg, then the front of the thigh. After rotating the kneecap, you use one thumb to press the point below the knee, the other to press down the inside shin. Stretch the foot forward and back, then repeat the sequence on the other leg.

The Back

The main meridian on the back is the Bladder Meridian, the longest in the body. This covers more than just the urinary function, since it is the *yang* aspect of the Water element in the body, covering all the related associations of reproduction, stamina, bones, teeth and head hair. The most important aspect of your back shiatsu is that you are stimulating the spinal nerves which supply all the internal organs. Almost every *tsubo* on the Bladder Meridian on the back directly influences the supply of *ki* energy to another meridian. The points at the top influence the lungs and heart; the *tsubos* on the middle back affect the organs concerned with digestion – the left-hand side relating mainly to the stomach, the right to the liver and gall bladder; the lumbar area is connected with the kidneys and the large and small intestines; while the sacrum connects with the bladder itself. With practice it is possible to diagnose a great deal about the internal functions simply by feeling the state of the spine and the surrounding musculature. But in the beginning, it is not necessary to have an exact knowledge of the correspondences. Just working thoroughly down the spine will balance the *ki* naturally, as long as you are sensitive to your partner's reactions.

Back Map

The back reflects the condition of the internal energies in its structure. The areas for the Lungs, Heart Protector (emotions and circulation) and Heart lie between the shoulderblades. The Stomach and Triple Heater are on the left of the middle back, the Liver and Gall Bladder on the right. The Spleen affects a small area around the twelfth thoracic vertebra. The Kidneys and Intestines dominate the lumbar area and the sacrum reflects the Bladder. Problem areas in the back may indicate trouble in the corresponding organ function.

Key to the Meridians

Bl	*Bladder*	**GB**	*Gall Bladder*
Ki	*Kidney*	**SI**	*Small Intestine*
Liv	*Liver*	**LI**	*Large Intestine*
St	*Stomach*	**TH**	*Triple Heater*
Sp	*Spleen*	**HP**	*Heart Protector*
Ht	*Heart*	**GV**	*Governing Vessel*
Lu	*Lungs*	**CV**	*Conception Vessel*

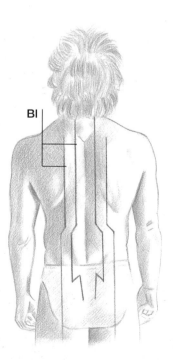

Back Meridians

The main meridian on the back is the Bladder Meridian, which is the largest in the body. It runs down each side of the vertebral column to the sacral area, where it turns twice, then reappears at the top of the back to form an "outer Bladder Meridian" parallel to the first. The inner meridian has more of a physical effect, while the outer mainly influences the mind and emotions.

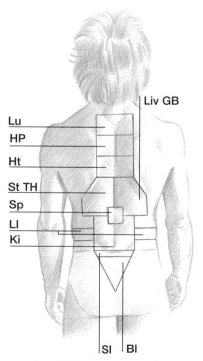

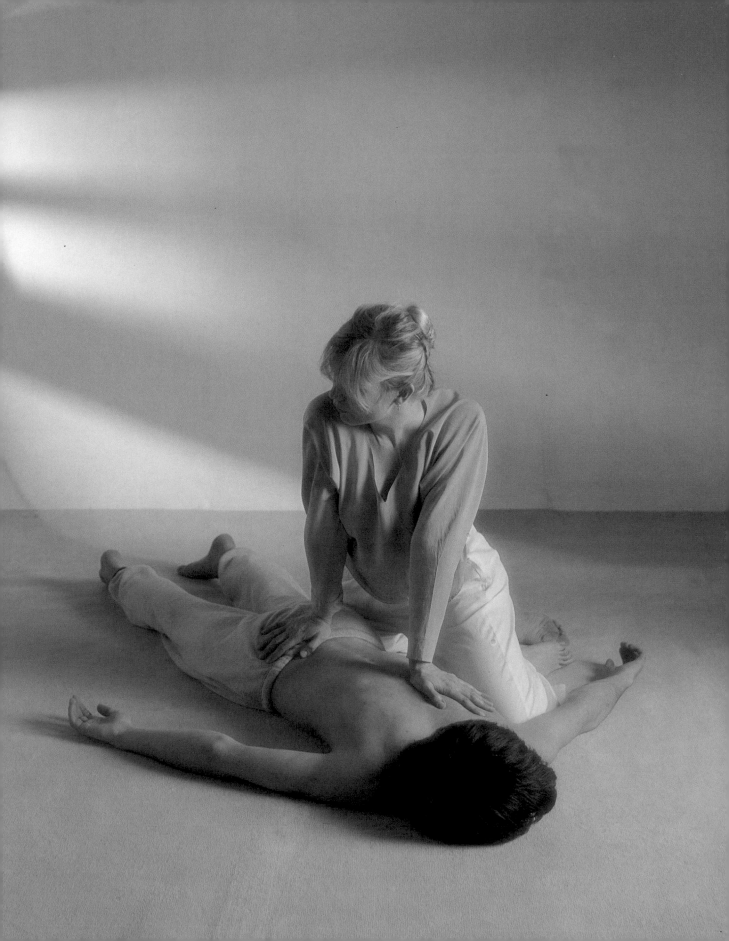

Diagonal Stretch

You begin a shiatsu treatment with the receiver lying on his or her front, arms by the sides, so that the spine receives maximum support. In this sequence of movements you are using your body weight to stretch the back. Keeping your knees apart, you kneel down beside your partner and place your hands diagonally on one shoulderblade and the opposite hip, hands facing away from one another and fingers splayed to increase your grip. The hip and shoulderblade act as natural "handles" with which to stretch the spine as you bring your own hips up and over. To begin with, repeat this sequence until you start to find your own working rhythm, keeping your movements slow enough for your partner to relax. As you become more practised, try to synchronize your pressure with your partner's outbreath – either by saying "breathe out" as you bring your hips forward, or by observing your partner's breathing pattern and harmonizing your movements with it. Working with the breathing is important – not only for the rhythm of your shiatsu but to help move the *ki* energy to where it needs to go.

Note: In our illustrations the giver is wearing a tight-fitting body suit for the sake of clarity only. To give shiatsu you must wear loose clothes.

1 Diagonal Stretch

A *Place one hand on your partner's shoulderblade, the other on the opposite hip, arms straight and fingers pointing in opposite directions. Now bring your hips up and forward so that you stretch your partner's back. Repeat once.*

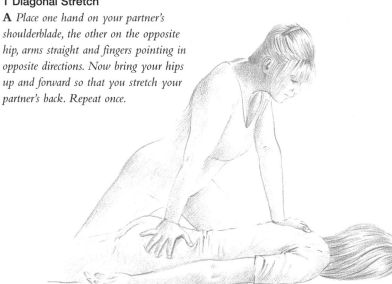

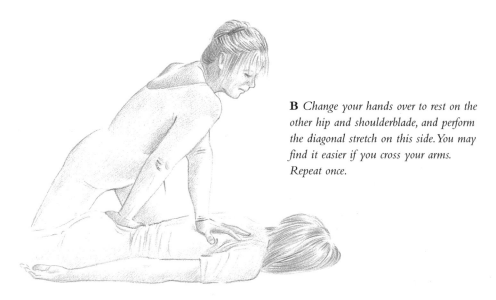

B *Change your hands over to rest on the other hip and shoulderblade, and perform the diagonal stretch on this side. You may find it easier if you cross your arms. Repeat once.*

Lumbar Stretch and Pressure down Spine

The lumbar stretch is an excellent movement for people with lower back problems, as it stretches the whole lumbar region. After repeating it two or three times you can begin to press down the Bladder Meridian beside the spine. You should start at the point on the shoulders where the back first runs horizontal. If you start your pressures on the downward slope of the upper shoulders, you will only push the flesh forward and will accomplish nothing. Don't go too fast – each pressure should last about three seconds or so. Work more lightly on the lumbar area; if the receiver has "disc trouble", avoid that immediate area and work above or below it. Ask your partner for feedback. Your pressure should feel good – if it hurts, it should be a "good hurt". Controlling the forward movement of your hips will moderate the amount of pressure you apply. In general you should work more on weak or hollow areas, less on tense or contracted ones. Make sure that your partner is not holding his or her breath. When you compress the back, synchronize your pressure with an exhalation.

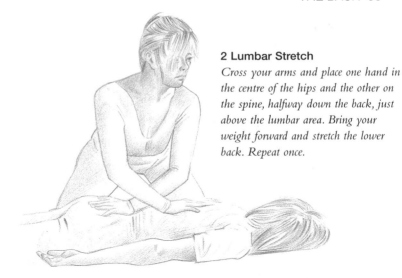

2 Lumbar Stretch

Cross your arms and place one hand in the centre of the hips and the other on the spine, halfway down the back, just above the lumbar area. Bring your weight forward and stretch the lower back. Repeat once.

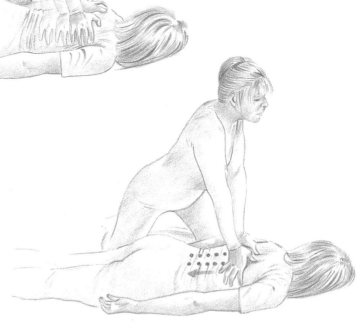

3 Palm Pressure down Spine

Place your hands on either side of the spine, halfway down the shoulders, heels alongside the spine and palms on the ribs. Bring your hips up and forward, transferring your weight through straight arms to your partner's back. Sit back and move your palms down a couple of centimetres (1 inch) or so, then repeat. Keep inching your way down until you reach the slope of the hips.

4 Thumb Pressure down Spine

Rest your fingers on the ribs and place your thumbs either side of the spine, halfway down the shoulders, making sure that they are not lying painfully on a bone. Then proceed as above, supporting most of your body on your thumbs but allowing your fingers to take a little of your weight. Move down a couple of centimetres (1 inch) at a time, applying pressure by bringing your hips forward, releasing it by moving them back.

The Hips

From a structural point of view, the hips are a complex area, since they are the junction point between the main mass of the body and its primary means of support and transport, the legs. Structural imbalance in the hips often results from lack of coordination between the legs and the axis of the spine – as when one leg is shorter than the other or when the spine is twisted to the left or right – and this causes low back pain or discomfort in the pelvic area. The basic drives of anger and sexuality also stem from the hips, for anger involves the kicking and stamping reflex and sexuality presupposes free movement of the pelvis. The lower back and buttocks may become tense and painful as a result of long-term repression of either of these instincts, or simply from the unnaturally sedentary lives many of us lead. The Bladder Meridian is the chief meridian on the hips – as it is on the back. The Gall Bladder Meridian on the side of each buttock has a major point slightly behind and above where the hip bone juts out. Giving shiatsu here can be very helpful for relieving low back pain or sciatica, but don't press too hard or you may inflame the sciatic nerve. Shiatsu to the hips also releases tension in the lumbar area, and relieves menstrual pain and cystitis and all kinds of congestion or pain in the pelvis. It is extremely soothing and relaxing, especially for women, who are more susceptible to pelvic congestion than men.

Hip Meridians
The outer and inner Bladder Meridians cover most of the sacrum and surrounding muscles. The Gall Bladder Meridian runs down the outside of the hips, passing over the sciatic nerve in the centre of the side of the buttocks.

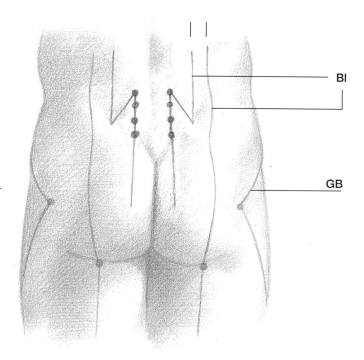

Bl

GB

See Key to Meridians on p. 92.

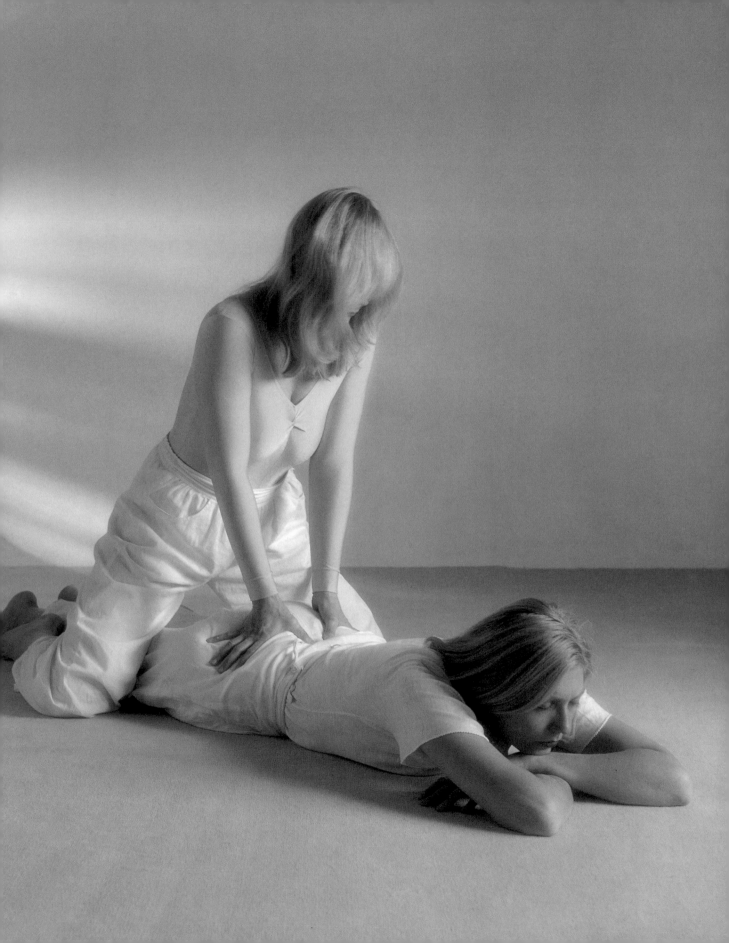

Hips (II)

Treating the hips begins with pressure on the four pairs of holes in the sacrum (shown right), through which you contact the spinal nerves supplying the pelvis. It is often hard to locate these holes at first. Look for the softer areas in the bony triangle at the base of the spine, getting feedback from your partner as to what feels good. The two upper pairs appear as softer hollows in the hard surround; the two lower ones may be difficult to find even after years of experience, but persevere. Using your elbow on the buttocks also takes practice, but if you keep your centre of gravity low and your hand relaxed, you will find your elbow a useful tool. The meridians that you are treating are extensions of the Bladder Meridian: one goes down about 4 cm (1½ inches) on either side of the division between the buttocks, the other is on the highest point of the curve in the centre of the buttocks.

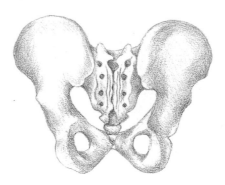

Locating the Sacral Holes

The sacrum is the bony triangle at the base of the vertebral column. Locating the outline of this triangle will help you to find the four pairs of hollows, or foramina, in the sacrum, through which the spinal nerves pass. If your partner has dimples on the hips, the top pair of tsubos *usually lies just within them.*

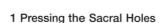

1 Pressing the Sacral Holes

Kneel astride your partner's legs. Locate the upper pair of holes with your thumbs. Now bring your hips forward and "lean" into the holes. Move your weight back and locate the pair of holes about 2–3 cm (1 inch) below. Leaning forward, press into these. The two lowest pairs are harder to locate. Use your intuition and "lean" into where you think they are.

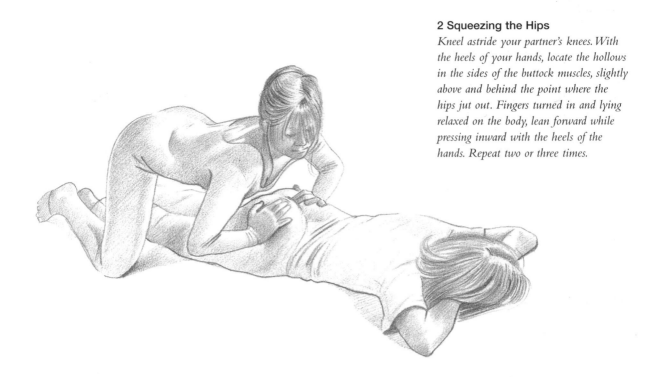

2 Squeezing the Hips

Kneel astride your partner's knees. With the heels of your hands, locate the hollows in the sides of the buttock muscles, slightly above and behind the point where the hips jut out. Fingers turned in and lying relaxed on the body, lean forward while pressing inward with the heels of the hands. Repeat two or three times.

3 Elbow Pressure down Hips

Knees wide apart, place one hand on the small of the back for support. Keeping the other hand relaxed, lay your "open" elbow on the meridian line close to the division of the buttocks. Lean forward and bring the weight of your upper body on to your elbow. Proceed in this way down both meridians on both sides. Don't use a sharp, "closed" elbow or allow your hands to tense up during the treatment.

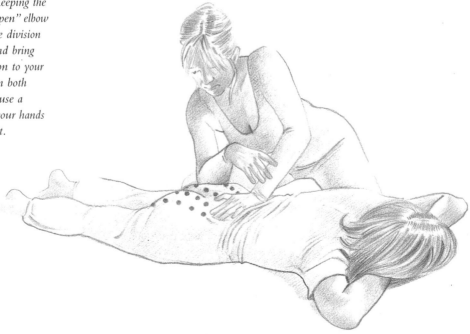

Back and Outside of Legs

The main meridians on the back of the leg – the Bladder Meridian and its paired meridian, the Kidney Meridian – belong to the Water element (p. 83). The Bladder Meridian continues down the legs from the spine and the Kidney ascends through important postural muscles which connect with the pelvis and lower back, so that the back of the leg is a useful area for treating lower backache. The Bladder and Kidneys and their meridians represent respectively the *yang* and *yin* aspects of the Water element, which governs genetic inheritance and growth, repro-duction, sexual energy and the individual's basic constitution. The Gall Bladder Meridian traverses the outside of the leg. The Gall Bladder is the *yang* aspect of Wood, which governs the eyes and rules over the tendons and the contractile quality of muscles, as well as contributing to the process of digestion. Emotional and mental stress affect the Wood element in much the same way as the abuse of the body affects the Water element. The Gall Bladder tends to react more to mental strain, decision-making and work worries, while its paired function, the Liver, is more affected by emotional factors. Mental strain affecting the meridian is likely to bring on tension in the neck and shoulders, headaches and even migraines, since the Gall Bladder Meridian traverses the neck, shoulders and sides of the head. While it is obviously beneficial to work on the affected areas, in practice you can treat these conditions by working on the side of the leg to keep the *ki* energy circulating freely through the whole meridian.

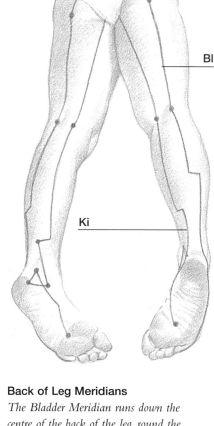

Back of Leg Meridians

The Bladder Meridian runs down the centre of the back of the leg, round the outside of the ankle and down the foot to the little toe. The Kidney Meridian starts on the sole, loops around the inner heel, then runs up between the muscles of the inner calf and thigh.

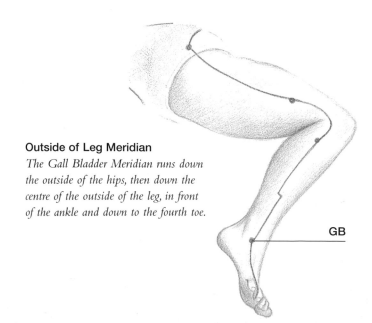

Outside of Leg Meridian

The Gall Bladder Meridian runs down the outside of the hips, then down the centre of the outside of the leg, in front of the ankle and down to the fourth toe.

See Key to Meridians on p. 92.

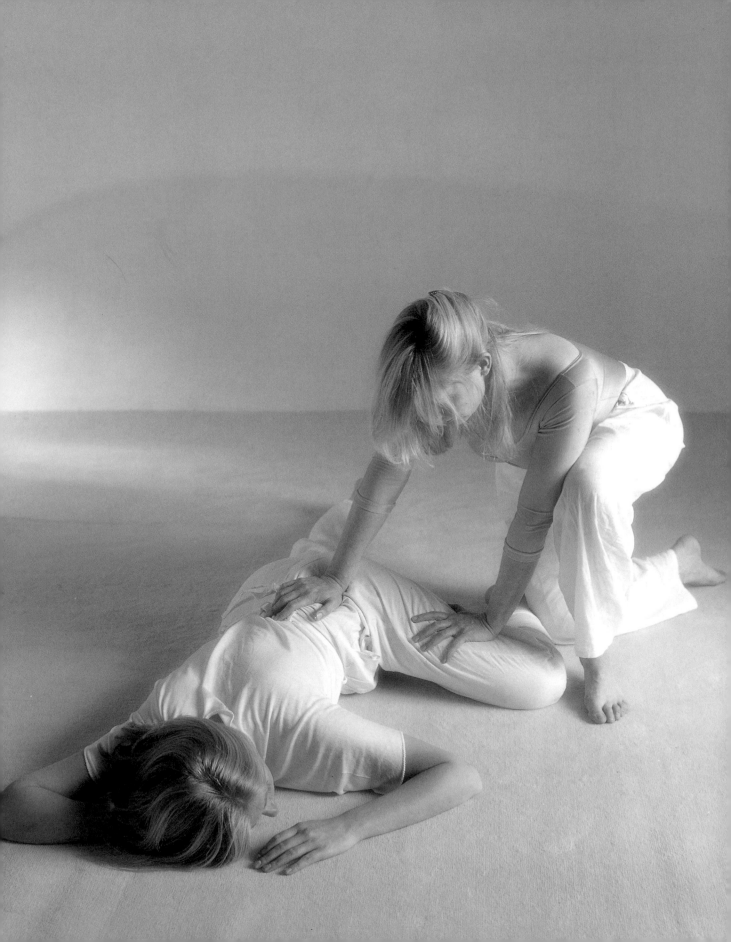

Back and Outside of Legs (II)

In this series of movements you work on the back and side of the leg in one unbroken sequence. Stay with the same leg until you have covered both back and side meridians. Your partner's feet should be lying flat and slightly pigeon-toed, unless this is uncomfortable. If the knees are painful or the ankles stiff, place a pillow under the shins to ease the pressure. Be careful not to press on the backs of the knees during this sequence and use less pressure on both sides of the area. Whenever you give shiatsu, both hands remain in contact with the body. When you are working on a limb, you should keep one hand on the torso, to maintain a connection with the main energy source. This hand, known as the "mother" hand, is supportive and static, while the other is active, like a child which runs about but continually comes back to its mother and draws nourishment from her. The exact positioning of the "mother" hand is not important, since it does not apply pressure. But you should remain conscious of it, using it to "listen" for reactions from your partner.

1 Palm Pressure on Back of Leg
Kneeling parallel to the receiver's leg, press down the centre of the leg with your palm or the "dragon's mouth" hold, using your body weight. Keep your "mother" hand on the buttock and press very lightly on the back of the knee and moderately on the calf. As you approach the ankle, squeeze gently as well as pressing. Repeat once.

2 Knee Pressure on Back of Leg
Support yourself with your hands at the top and bottom of the leg. Squat on tiptoe, keeping your knees above the leg's midline. Now lightly "bounce" your knees up and down the centre of the leg, avoiding the knee area. Don't kneel on the leg – you should be able to drop your knee on to it as lightly or heavily as you wish.

3 Pressing Ankle *Tsubos*
Lift the foot of the same leg and press both sides of the hollow between the ankle bone and the Achilles tendon for about 3–5 seconds.

Three-way Stretch

This sequence works on the meridians at the front and sides of the leg, although you are applying shiatsu from the back. Stretch the leg in each direction as far as is comfortable for your partner. After completing the three movements, rearrange your partner's position so that you can go straight on to work on the side of the leg.

Caution: Do not do the Three-way Stretch on anyone with knee problems.

4 Three-way Stretch

A *With one hand on the small of the back, use the other to bring the foot back toward the buttock, holding the foot under the toes for maximum stretch. Bounce the foot a little at the point of maximum extension.*

B *Take the foot halfway back to release the knee. Then bring it over to the opposite buttock, as far as it will comfortably go. Bounce it up and down a little to increase the stretch.*

C *Take the foot halfway back once more. Then bring it over toward you as far as it will go. Bounce it up and down again. Now take it halfway back, without releasing the foot. With your other hand, pick up the inside of the knee and crook the leg outward, ready for Palm Pressure down Side of Leg, as shown on page 104.*

Back and Outside of Legs (III)

Pressing down the side of the leg with your palms completes the sequence on the leg. Don't be afraid to crook your partner's leg right out to the side – it is more comfortable than it looks. After working right down the leg, straighten it out again and repeat the whole sequence on the other leg, before beginning on the feet. With the feet, too, you run through the entire series of movements on one foot, then change to the other. Walking on the soles not only feels great to your partner, it also gives you a rest. Most of the foot routine given here stimulates the Kidney and Bladder Meridians. Each meridian ends in a toe, so it is important to pull your partner's toes thoroughly.

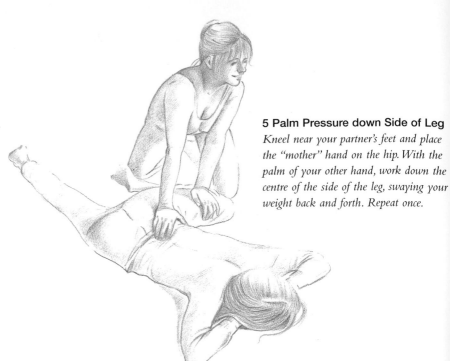

5 Palm Pressure down Side of Leg
Kneel near your partner's feet and place the "mother" hand on the hip. With the palm of your other hand, work down the centre of the side of the leg, swaying your weight back and forth. Repeat once.

6 Pressing Ankle *Tsubo*
With your thumb, press the sensitive hollow just below and slightly to the front of the outside ankle bone for 3–5 seconds.

Repeat 1–6 on the other leg.

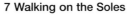

7 Walking on the Soles
Making sure both your partner's feet are lying as flat on the ground as possible, walk your feet up and down on the soles for a minute or two. Don't let your feet go too high up the instep.

8 Pressing *Tsubo* on Sole
Use your thumb to press the Kidney point under the ball of the foot, in the centre, for 3–5 seconds.

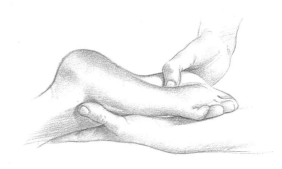

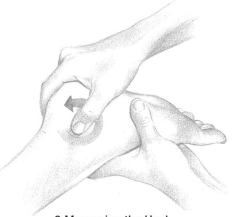

9 Massaging the Heel
Massage the sides of the heel with a circular movement, thumb on one side, fingers on the other, for 5–10 seconds.

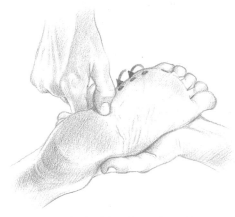

10 Pinching Outside of Foot
Pinch along the outside edge of the foot, to stimulate the Bladder Meridian.

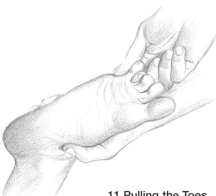

11 Pulling the Toes
Use a firm tugging movement to pull each toe in turn, holding it at the side, for that is where the nerves are. Some toes may crack when tension is released.

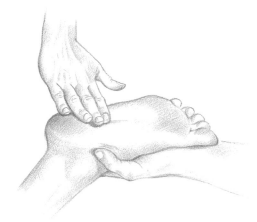

12 Slapping the Sole
Keeping your wrist relaxed so that your hand can flap up and down freely, slap the sole repeatedly in a fast, forceful rhythm.

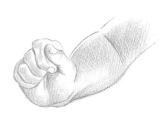

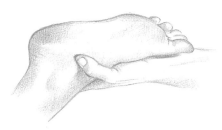

13 Pounding the Sole
Use the same wrist movement to pound the sole of the foot for a few seconds, with your hand in a relaxed fist. Then stroke the foot to soothe it.

Repeat 8–13 on the other foot.

Back of Shoulders

Now comes the back of the shoulders, where tension is an almost universal problem. However, this tension can come from any one of many causes, perhaps originating in other parts of the body, so don't be tempted to give shiatsu to the shoulders only. The problem will soon return unless you locate and treat the cause during a full body treatment. There are three main areas to treat on the back of the shoulders. The first is the top of the shoulders, which is connected to the Gall Bladder Meridian. Since the Gall Bladder relates to mental stress, this area is nearly always tender. Besides relieving stress, it is also good for treating colds and headaches. The second area is the central part of the shoulders, between the blades. This is the part of the Bladder Meridian which you left out when treating the rest of the back, because it was sloping away from you (see p. 95). The uppermost points are good for colds, coughs and any lung problems; the lower ones affect the heart and circulation and are also good for anxiety, distress, and insomnia. The shoulderblades themselves constitute the third area, crossed by the Small Intestine Meridian, which is concerned with digestion, with ovarian function in women and with the mental function of intuitive clarity. You will be treating the neck later, after your partner turns over, but massage the neck muscles occasionally if they get stiff.

Back of Shoulder Anatomy
The tsubos of the Bladder Meridian lie between the vertebrae on each side of the spine, and down the edges of the shoulderblades. The Small Intestine Meridian runs through the thick covering of muscle over the shoulderblade, while the Gall Bladder Meridian travels along the ridge of muscle at the top.

Back of Shoulder Meridians
The Bladder Meridian runs down the sides of the spine and the Gall Bladder Meridian across the top of the shoulder. The Small Intestine Meridian zigzags across the shoulderblade and down the back of the arm, alongside the Triple Heater.

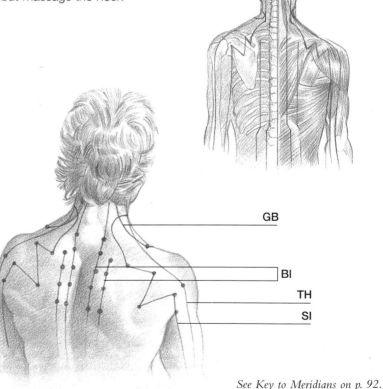

GB

BI

TH

SI

See Key to Meridians on p. 92.

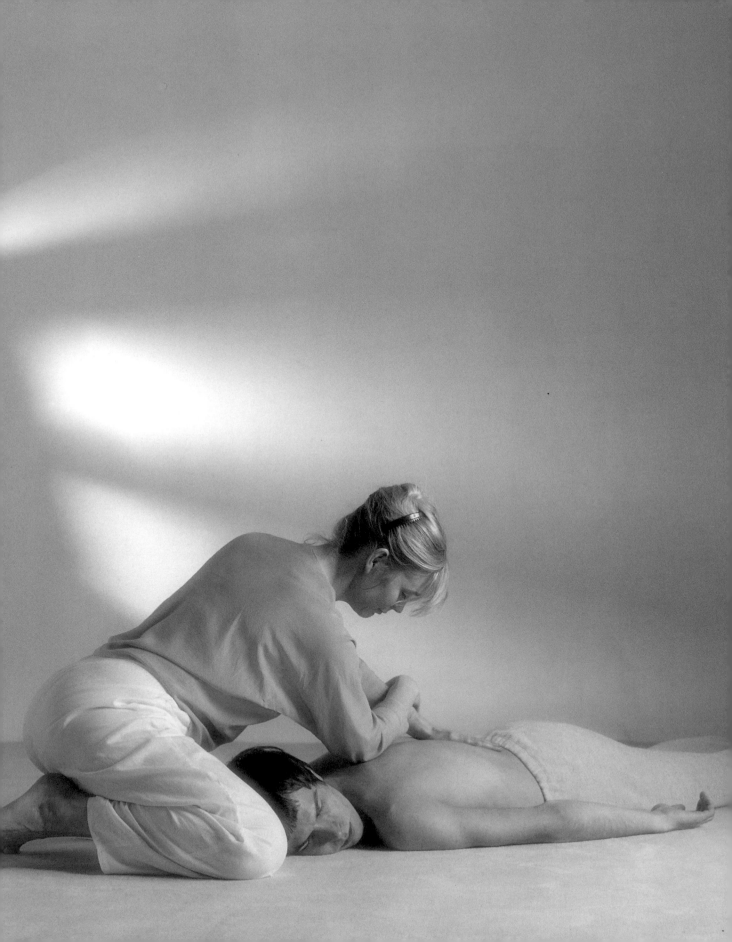

Back of Shoulders (II)

You now move up to kneel slightly astride your partner's head. In this sequence you don't lift your hips up and forward, as this would put too much weight on your partner. But your pressure should still come from the hips, since you lean forward and allow your partner to support the top part of your body. You start by treating the ridge of muscles along the top of the shoulders, which is often tender with tension. Then use your elbow to work down between the shoulderblades to affect the lungs and heart. The whole of this central area is closely linked with emotions and consciousness, so you should treat it with respect, working gently but deeply. The Small Intestine Meridian, which zigzags across each shoulderblade, is hard to locate precisely, so you treat it by rotating the shoulderblades to loosen the muscles and release the energy locked in them. Often there is a contradictory situation of tense, tight muscles covering low basic energy. Be gentle, making up for your lack of force by the duration of your pressure, and the muscles will relax.

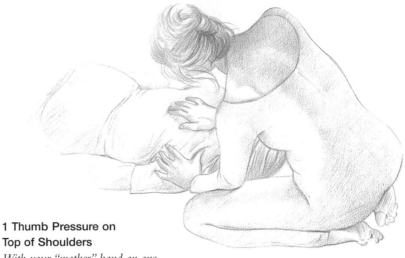

1 Thumb Pressure on Top of Shoulders

With your "mother" hand on one shoulderblade, lay the length of the thumb of the other hand along the top of one shoulder. Rest your elbow on your thigh for support. Leaning forward, press gently out from the neck to the notch in the shoulder joint, three times each side, as detailed right.

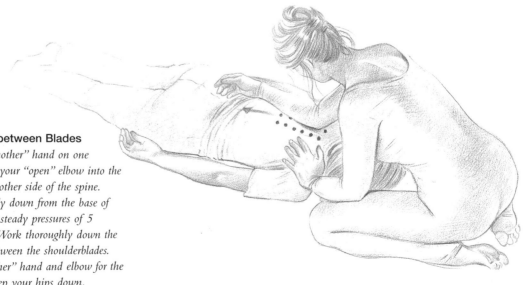

2 Elbowing between Blades

With your "mother" hand on one shoulder, lean your "open" elbow into the groove on the other side of the spine. Work gradually down from the base of the neck with steady pressures of 5 seconds or so. Work thoroughly down the whole area between the shoulderblades. Change "mother" hand and elbow for the other side. Keep your hips down.

3 Rotating the Shoulderblades

Place both your hands flat on your partner's shoulderblades, fingers spread to give you a better grip. Curl your fingers under the outside of the blades and rotate them firmly, moving the shoulderblades themselves and also the muscles above and below them.

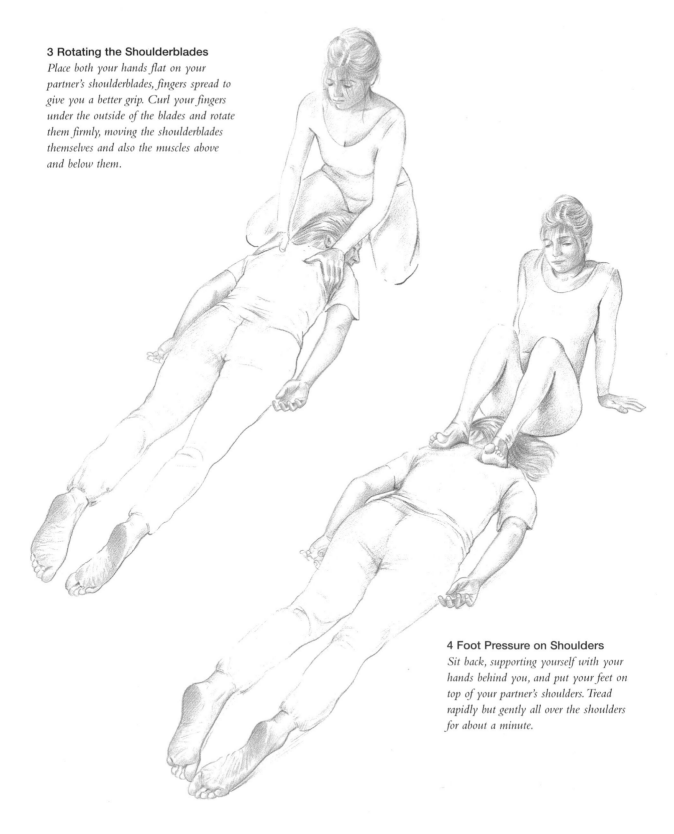

4 Foot Pressure on Shoulders

Sit back, supporting yourself with your hands behind you, and put your feet on top of your partner's shoulders. Tread rapidly but gently all over the shoulders for about a minute.

Front of Shoulders and Neck

Shiatsu on the front of the body begins with the shoulders and neck. Weakness at the front of the shoulders often causes tight or tense muscles at the back – a classic example of a *kyo*, or deficient condition, creating a *jitsu* or excess one. And frequently, stooped or rounded shoulders result from an instinctive hunching to protect a weak chest or, occasionally, to protect an over-vulnerable "heart" centre. These conditions can be worked on most effectively from the front. You start your treatment by leaning on your partner's shoulders, where your pressure falls mainly on the Lung points, then work outward between the ribs. Having opened up the chest and straightened the shoulders, you then move up to treat the neck, working first on the Bladder Meridian, next on the Gall Bladder, then on the Governing Vessel and, finally, pressing important points on all the neck meridians along the base of the skull. The meridians of the Triple Heater, Small Intestine, Large Intestine and Stomach cover the sides and front of the neck, making it an area very much connected with the digestive function – and, indeed, the throat is one of the uppermost parts of the digestive tract. Since each meridian has a psychological function as well as a physical one, these meridians also deal with "digesting" information and events. When life presents us with something we cannot "swallow" or "stomach", it creates tension in the throat and neck muscles, as well as affecting the digestion. Shiatsu to this area involves a gentle rotation of the muscles, rather than direct pressure which might damage the windpipe or arteries.

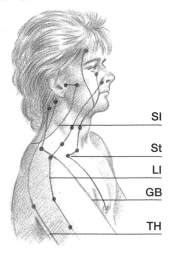

SI
St
LI
GB
TH

Side of Neck Meridians
The Stomach Meridian runs down each side of the windpipe, while the Large Intestine crosses the centre of the muscle at the side of the neck and goes down into the sensitive nerve plexus above the collarbone. The Small Intestine runs directly down from the ear, with the Triple Heater slightly behind it.

Back of Neck Meridians
The central meridian is the Governing Vessel, which runs up the middle of the vertebral column. The Bladder Meridian passes down the centre of the muscles on either side of the neck, while the Gall Bladder runs down the outer edge of the same muscles.

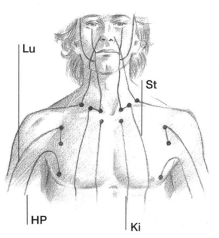

Lu

St

HP

Ki

Front of Shoulder Meridians
Important points at the start of the Lung Meridian lie in the hollow under the outer portion of the collarbone. The Heart Protector lies along the pectoral muscle, and the Stomach and Kidney pass down the front of the chest.

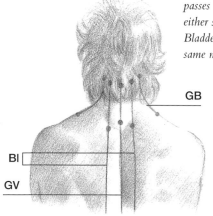

GB

BI

GV

See Key to Meridians on p. 92.

Front of Shoulders and Neck

Your partner now turns over and you resume your kneeling position on either side of the head, to lean on the front of the shoulders and press along between the ribs. When leaning on the front of the shoulders, your main pressure falls on the Lung points in the hollows between the chest and the shoulder joints. Then, as you work outward between the ribs, you not only stretch the intercostal muscles which assist with breathing, but also activate the Kidney and Stomach Meridians which increase *ki* energy in the chest and help to eliminate phlegm. Shiatsu to this area is very helpful for asthmatics. Use your body weight to lean on the shoulders and open the chest, but exert less pressure when working on the sensitive spaces between the ribs.

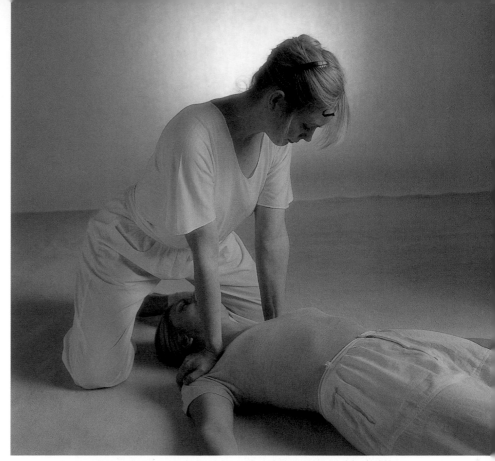

1 Leaning on the Shoulders

Place the heels of your hands in the hollows between your partner's chest and shoulder joints, fingers turned outward, enclosing the rounded part of the shoulders. Now bring your hips up and forward and lean on the shoulders, as above right.

2 Pressing along the Ribs

Place your hands so that the palms face down the sides of the body and the thumbs rest along the front of the chest, in a space between two ribs. Lean forward slightly and press gently, with the whole length of the thumb, outward from the breastbone. Now move to the space between the next two ribs and cover the whole upper chest in this way. Avoid the breasts when working with a female partner.

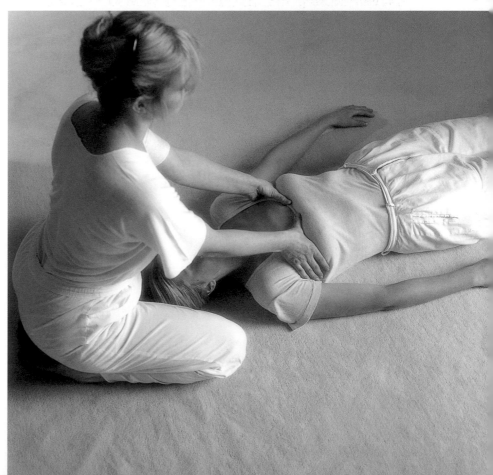

The Neck

Treating the neck from underneath rather than above is far more convenient, because the neck is straight and your partner therefore more relaxed. The only problem is to achieve firm pressure without lifting your partner's head away from the ground. As always in shiatsu, the answer is to position yourself as illustrated right so that your pressure comes "from the *hara*". The first meridian you work on is the Bladder, up either side of the spine at the back of the neck. The second is the Gall Bladder, which lies in the seam between the two muscles, and is extremely useful for relieving stiff necks, tension headaches and eye problems. A major point lies on this meridian in the hollow at the base of the skull on each side, which clears the head and alleviates cold symptoms. Third, you work up the Governing Vessel in the centre, which helps to realign the vertebrae, pressing gently in the central hollow at the base of the skull to stimulate the midbrain. And finally you move out along the base of the skull, pressing important points on all the meridians.

3 Neck Sequence

Knees on either side of your partner's head, rest your elbows on your thighs and lean forward from the hips, as you press upward with your fingers.

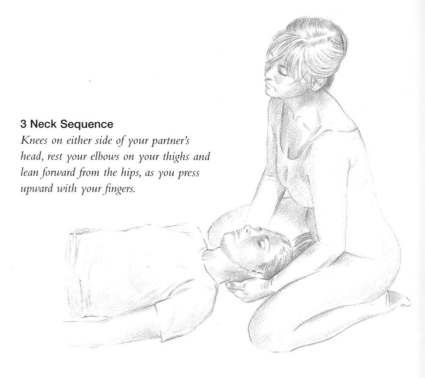

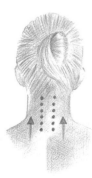

A *Using your middle fingers, press on either side of the spine at 1.5-cm (½-inch) intervals from the base of the neck upward to the base of the skull.*

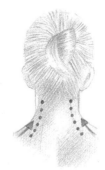

B *Move your fingers out to the outer edge of the large muscles at the back of the neck. Press at 1.5-cm (½-inch) intervals from the base of the neck up, applying more pressure in the hollows at the base of the skull. Repeat once.*

C *Go back to the midline of the neck and with your middle fingers on top of one another, press in the sensitive hollows between the vertebrae. Finish at the central hollow at the base of the skull.*

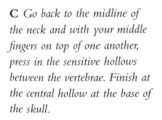

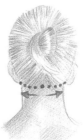

D *Separate your fingers and press firmly outward along the base of the skull toward the ears at 1.5-cm (½-inch) intervals.*

Sides of Neck

Several meridians run down the sides
of the neck and imbalances in these
are often a source of neck tension. But
since this area includes nerves
affecting the windpipe and a main
artery, it is better to stimulate the
meridians with a gentle circling
movement rather than direct pressure.
Stretching the neck is very beneficial
and releases tension in the vertebrae.
But be sure to hold your partner's
head firmly and use your body weight
to stretch backward, not upward.

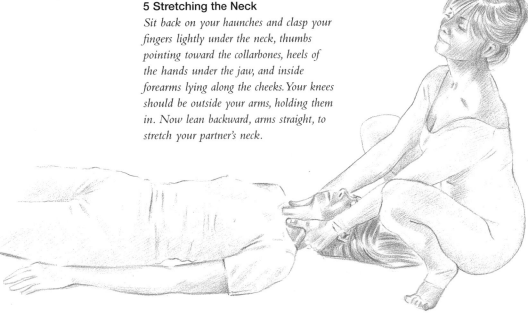

4 Circling Sides of Neck

*Lay your fingers close together on the
sides of your partner's neck, moulding
them to the curves of the neck. Now circle
slowly several times, moving the flesh over
the underlying muscles.*

5 Stretching the Neck

*Sit back on your haunches and clasp your
fingers lightly under the neck, thumbs
pointing toward the collarbones, heels of
the hands under the jaw, and inside
forearms lying along the cheeks. Your knees
should be outside your arms, holding them
in. Now lean backward, arms straight, to
stretch your partner's neck.*

Head and Face

For many people this is the most soothing and relaxing part of the treatment. We all have a tendency to "live in our heads", building up excess energy and tension there; and so many meridians begin and end on the face that blockages can easily occur, resulting in lines, blemishes, or sagging flesh as well as in more serious conditions. Shiatsu to this area removes any obstructions and increases the supply of *ki*, thus releasing tension and, as a happy side-effect, beautifying. As the late shiatsu master Shizuto Masunaga once said in his inimitable English: "Shiatsu to face is not only good for soul but make very beauty!" The meridians which begin on the head and face are the Bladder, Gall Bladder and Stomach, while those which end there are the Governing Vessel, Conception Vessel, Large Intestine, Small Intestine and Triple Heater. If your partner suffers from migraines, you may wish to pay special attention to the sides of the head – the Gall Bladder Meridian doubles back on itself several times to cover each side. Our shiatsu sequence for the head and face consists mainly of pressure on key points rather than meridians. Face points are most often used to relieve local tension, pain or congestion. Their effect on the rest of the meridian is on the subtle energy level, rather than the physical one. Thus, a Bladder point near the eye will not affect the bladder although it will have a subtle effect on the *ki* of the Water element.

Front of Face Points

In the area of the eyes: Bladder 1 is in the inner corner of the eye socket, just above the corner of the eye; Bladder 2 is at the inner end of the eyebrow. Around the mouth: Large Intestine 20 is just below the widest part of the nostril; Stomach 3 lies halfway down the "laughter line"; Conception Vessel 24 is in the centre of the chin groove; and Governing Vessel 26 lies in the centre of the upper lip.

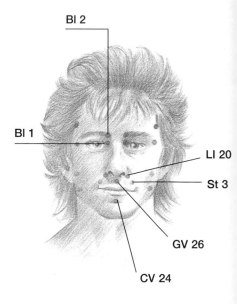

Top of Head Points

All these points lie on the Governing Vessel Meridian, and you cover them as you work along the midline of the head. The most important is Governing Vessel 20, which is on an imaginary line from the tops of the ears to the midline.

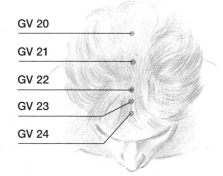

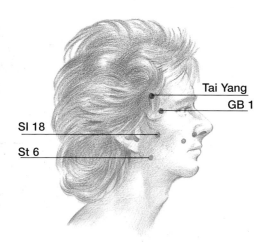

Side of Face Points

Tai Yang lies on the temple. Small Intestine 18 is in the hollow below the cheekbone, and Stomach 6 is in the knot of muscle within the angle of the jaw. Gall Bladder 1 is in a little hollow on the outside edge of the eye socket

See Key to Meridians on p. 92.

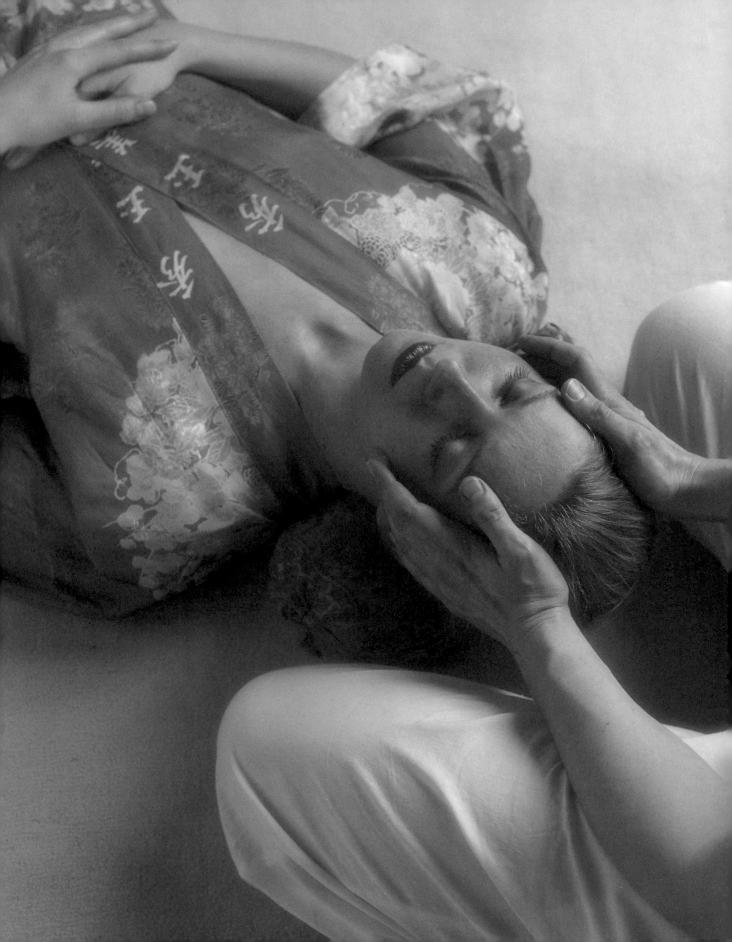

Head and Face (II)

Your shiatsu to this area should be gentle enough to relax your partner, but powerful enough to unblock energy. Keep the "feel" of your pressure firm but caressing and angle your fingers or thumbs when pressing points that lie in hollows or crevices. Massaging the ears benefits the whole person, since there are acupuncture points on the ear for each part of the body. The points on the top of the head are good for relieving headaches and nasal congestion. The eye sequence (opposite) not only benefits the eyes but also relieves headaches and sinus problems; the temple sequence is for general relaxation; and the nose-to-mouth sequence helps nasal and sinus congestion. It also releases emotional tension which may be expressed around the mouth, and can have a profoundly comforting effect.

1 Running Hands through Hair

Run your hands through your partner's hair a few times, so that your fingers brush the whole scalp, working back from the hairline.

2 Pulling the Hair

Taking one section of hair at a time, tug it gently. Pull lightly all over the head.

3 Massaging the Ears

Massage the ears between your thumbs and forefingers, moving up from the lobes to the tops of the ears. Cover the whole ear twice.

4 Pressing Top of Head Points

Hold your partner's head at the temples and, overlapping your thumbs on the midline of the head, press at 1.5-cm (½-inch) intervals back toward the crown as far as you can go.

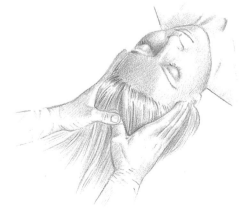

5 Eyes Sequence

A *Press the points at the inner corners of the eye sockets for 3–5 seconds.*

B *Pinch lightly along the length of the eyebrows.*

C *Press the points just outside the bony ridge at the outer end of each eyebrow.*

6 Temples Sequence

A *From the eyebrows, move up and out to the points on the temples. Don't press hard but rotate gently.*

B *Move down in a straight line to press the points just under the cheekbones.*

C *Move down in a straight line to the little knots of muscle just inside the angle of the jaw, and feel for the point in the centre of each knot. The sensation for the receiver is like toothache when you find it.*

7 Nose and Mouth Sequence

A *With the edge of your thumbs, press into the grooves beside the lower edge of the nostrils.*

B *Press the line of points along the "laughter lines", directing your pressure upward under the bone.*

C *Cup your hand under the chin and press the points in the centre of the groove of the chin and the centre of the upper lip.*

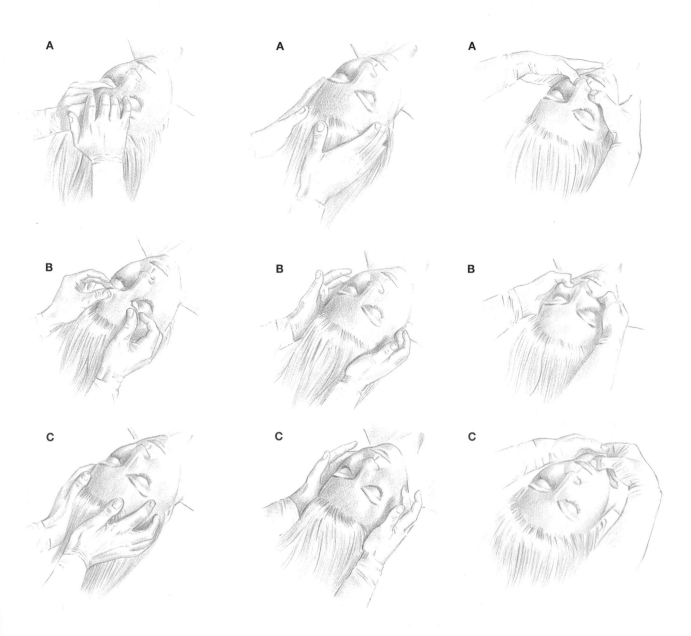

A   A   A

B   B   B

C   C   C

Arms and Hands

The six meridians in the arms and hands are those of the Fire and Metal elements. The Heart, Small Intestine, Heart Protector and Triple Heater Meridians belong to Fire, while the Lung and Large Intestine constitute Metal. The Oriental system considers the heart to be the house of the spirit, in addition to its known anatomical function of controlling the blood circulation. Anything to do with consciousness, such as mental disturbance, poor memory or insomnia, is related to the heart. Actual physical heart problems may involve either the Heart Meridian or, more often, the Heart Protector. The function of the Heart Protector is to act as a kind of buffer, shielding the heart from emotional stress; where it is weak, the heart is vulnerable to attack. As well as its physical function of digestion, the Small Intestine is concerned with the psychological functions of discrimination and awareness. The Triple Heater coordinates and balances the metabolism, acting on the "three burning spaces" – the upper, middle, and lower areas of the torso, which deal with circulation and respiration, digestion, and elimination respectively – and harmonizing their different spheres of activity. Fire is the only element with four functions; Metal has the normal complement of two – Lung and Large Intestine. The Lung acts as the receiver of *ki* from the air, and is thus concerned with the general level of *ki* energy as well as with lung and throat problems. The Large Intestine Meridian is not only concerned with the bowels; its province is elimination in general, through the skin and lungs in particular, so that acne or asthma can be Large Intestine problems. Since the meridian leads to the nose, it can also be helpful with sinus or nasal congestion.

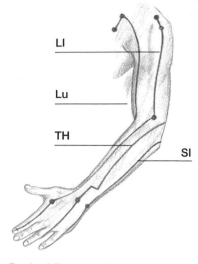

Back of Forearm Meridians
The Small Intestine continues down the outer edge of the forearm to the little finger. The Triple Heater travels down the centre to the ring finger, and the Large Intestine from the elbow crease to the forefinger.

Back of Upper Arm Meridians
The Small Intestine runs down the back of the arm from the armpit crease, the Triple Heater from the back of the shoulder to the "funny bone", and the Large Intestine down the top of the shoulder to the end of the elbow crease.

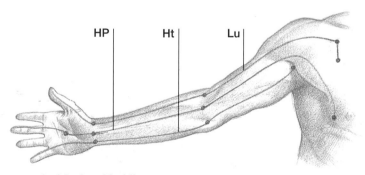

Inside Arm Meridians
The Lung Meridian runs from below the collarbone, down toward the thumb, the Heart Protector from the pectoral muscle down the arm toward the middle finger, and the Heart Meridian from the armpit to the little finger.

See Key to Meridians on p. 92.

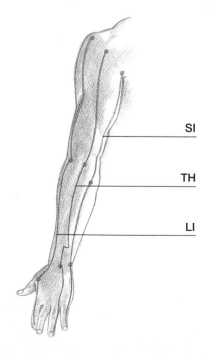

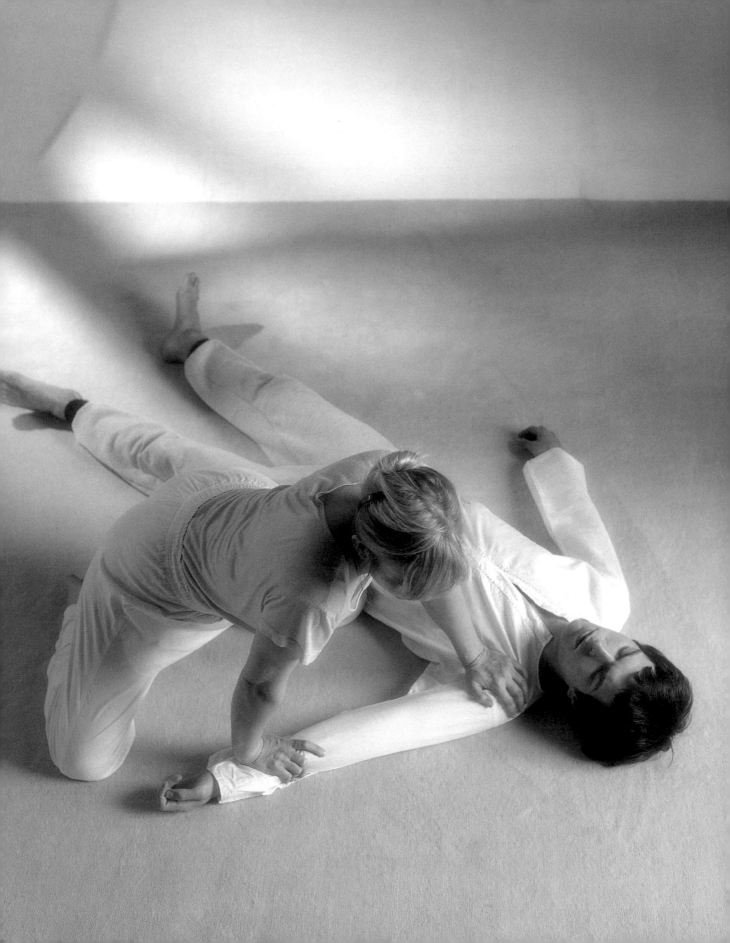

Arms and Hands (II)

Since it is a little complicated to treat all six arm meridians individually, in this sequence you learn to treat the arm in three stages – inner meridians, outer meridians and hand. Simple pressure down the whole arm is fine for the inner meridians. But because of a twist in the elbow joint, the outer meridians lie at the back of the arm above the elbow and at the front below it, so you must treat them in two stages, as shown below. The area just below the elbow is often painful when you press down the forearm, because of the nerve running underneath. Be sure to go right down to the wrist and press on the wrist joint – there are several key points on the wrist. Treat one arm at a time, completing all movements before moving yourself to the opposite side of your partner and giving shiatsu to the other arm and hand.

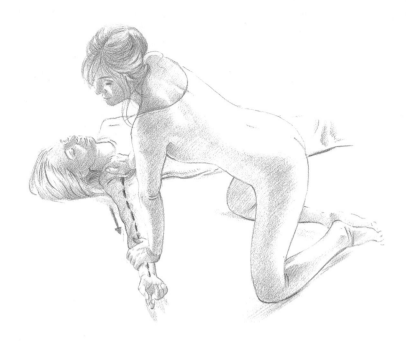

1 Palm Pressure along Inner Arm

Kneeling at your partner's hips, lay your partner's arm out horizontally from the shoulder, palm facing up. Place your "mother" hand on the pectoral muscle and apply palm pressure down the inner arm from shoulder to wrist. Mould your hand to the contours of the arm.

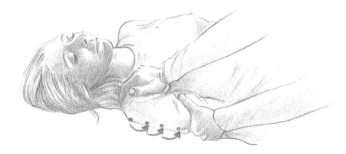

2 Grasping Upper Arm

Lay the arm down by your partner's side, palm facing down. With your "mother" hand on the shoulder, grasp the upper arm and apply pressure to the back of it with your fingertips, from shoulder to elbow.

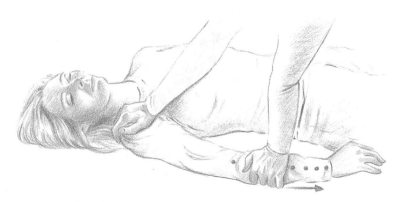

3 Palm Pressure down Forearm

Apply direct downward pressure to the forearm, from elbow to wrist.

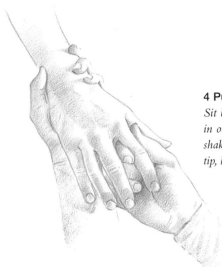

4 Pulling the Fingers

Sit back and take your partner's wrist in one hand. With the other, pull and shake each finger in turn, from base to tip, holding the finger at the sides.

5 Pressing the "Great Eliminator"

Press the point in the middle of the web of flesh between thumb and forefinger for 5 seconds. One of the most important points, this tsubo *on the Large Intestine Meridian was known as the "Great Eliminator" in ancient times. It helps specifically to eliminate headaches, toothaches, and colds.*

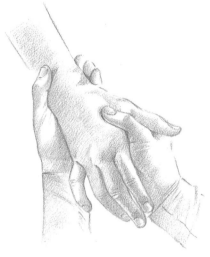

6 Shaking the Arm

Hold your partner's hand firmly in both of your own. Lean back until the arm is slightly stretched and shake it up and down, fast but not too vigorously.

Repeat 1–6 on the other arm.

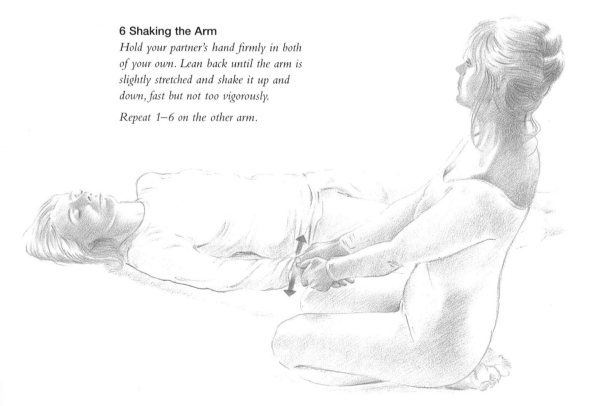

The *Hara*

To the Japanese, the *hara*, or abdomen, means far more than simply an area of the body. They consider that the vital spirit resides in the *hara*, more specifically at a point a hand's breadth below the navel, known as the "Tan-Den". In Japan, "*hara*" describes the quality of a person's energy – you may have a "good *hara*" or a "bad *hara*" and to kill yourself is to kill the *hara* – "*hara kiri*". Shiatsu to the *hara*, called *ampuku*, is a very ancient healing art – far older than shiatsu itself and requiring years of training. For a skilled practitioner of *ampuku* it is possible to treat and cure serious diseases working only on the *hara*. It is at the *hara* that all the vital processes of the body's support systems take place and that each of the meridian functions can be contacted. Like the foot in reflexology, the *hara* can be mapped out in reflex zones (as below) which reflect the state of all the body functions. So your work on the *hara* is a vitally important part of the treatment and, with experience, can become a valuable aid to diagnosis. Ideally, the *hara* should be soft and relaxed above the navel, and full and firm below it, but in practice, the average Western *hara* is quite the reverse. Sedentary living, poor eating and drinking habits, and lack of attention to breathing and posture contribute to universally weak conditions in the lower *hara* and Tan-Den, while mental and emotional strain lead to diaphragm tension and thus to a tight upper *hara*. Although you may not yet be able to diagnose these conditions by touch, you can assume that the lower *hara* is weak, and work first to strengthen it with deep, gradual, tonifying pressure before you proceed to the upper *hara*. This should have relaxed as you worked on the deficiency in the lower regions and you will be able to apply deeper pressure. When *ampuku* is done well and caringly, it is the most relaxing and comforting experience imaginable, benefiting and balancing all physical functions. It is especially good for abdominal problems and, above all, for the back. If your partner has a painful back condition, work thoroughly on the *hara*, particularly on the reflex area for the Bladder Meridian, before working on the back itself.

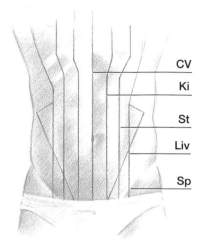

**Hara* Meridians*
Although you can affect the functioning of all the meridians via the hara, *not all the meridian lines cross it. When giving shiatsu, it is more important to understand the* hara *map of the reflex zones (below) than the meridians.*

**Hara* Map*
The ribs and pelvic bones form the natural borders of the hara. Within these borders, the reflex areas for the meridians roughly follow the placement of the organs. The main exceptions are the two "horseshoes" of the Bladder and Kidney zones. The Kidney zone crosses the source of vital energy, or Tan-Den, and the Bladder zone connects with the muscles that support the spine, linking it with the Bladder Meridian.

See Key to Meridians on p. 92.

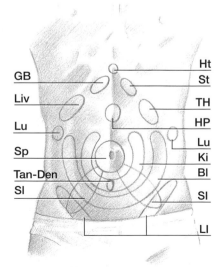

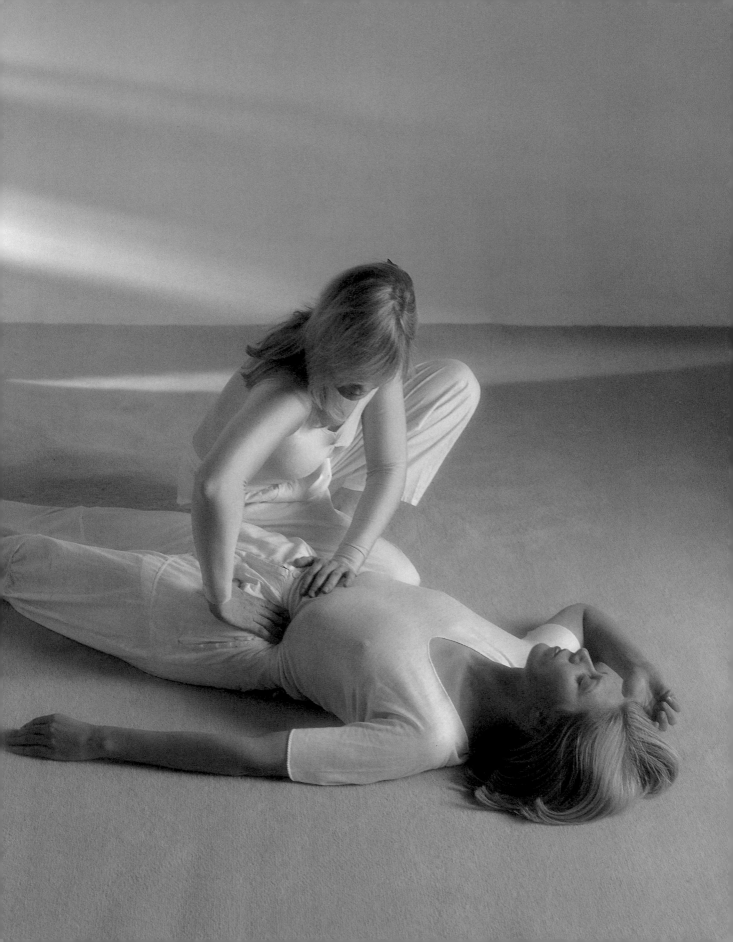

Hara (II)

As the official residence of the body's energies, the *hara* merits great respect. Even animals are reluctant to have their bellies touched, except by those they trust, and people are not so different. Your pressure should be very smooth and gradual, although it can be quite deep. Always work clockwise around the *hara*, strengthening the weaker areas with deep toning pressure before you work on tense, contracted ones. In most cases, this means starting on the lower *hara* (see p. 122). Keep your "mother" hand constantly in contact with the *hara* as you work, moving it whenever you need to and using it to "listen" for signs of change. Generally, a gurgle means that you have supplied a weak area with energy, a pulse that your pressure is creating an obstruction – except at the midline between ribs and navel, where a main artery runs and there is always a pulse.

Position for Working on the *Hara*

When giving ampuku, *or* shiatsu *to the* hara, *sit by your partner's side, with your thigh lightly touching theirs.*

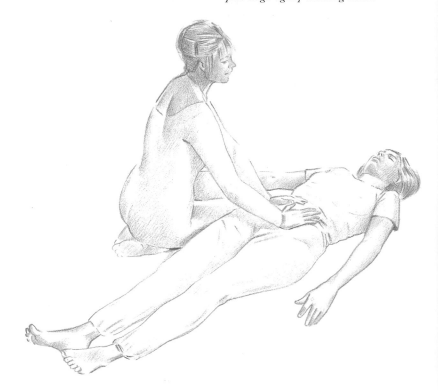

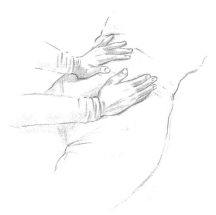

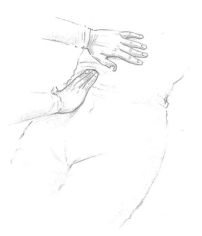

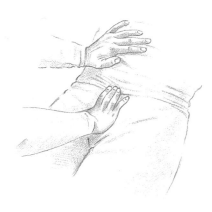

1 Lower *Hara*

A *Use the edge of your hand like a knife to go in beside the hip bones and work on the Large Intestine zone.*

B *With three fingers laid flat, press at 2–3-cm (1-inch) intervals clockwise around the outer horseshoe of the lower* hara, *to treat the Bladder zone.*

C *Work in the same way along the inner horseshoe, the semi-circular boundary of the central abdominal muscles, with longer pressure on the midline point. Here you are treating the Kidney zone and Tan-Den.*

2 Upper *Hara*

A *Press gently but deeply with the full length of your thumb under the left side of the ribs, working from top to bottom. Keep your palm and fingers in relaxed contact.*

B *With your fingertips, press inward in the hollow below the lowest point of the ribs – the Lung zone.*

C *Work in the same way down the right-hand side, ending with the same inward pressure under the ribs.*

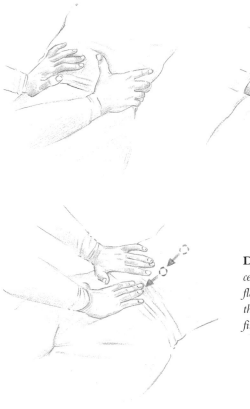

D *Press lightly with one finger under the central meeting of the ribs; then with three flat fingers on the solar plexus, halfway on the solar plexus, halfway to the navel; and finally on the navel area itself.*

3 Rocking the *Hara*

Move up and kneel facing your partner's hara. With one hand on top of the other, rock the hara with a wavelike motion, pushing with the heels of your hands and pulling toward you with the fingertips in one continuous movement.

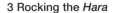

Front and Inside of Legs

There are three main meridians in this area – Liver, Spleen, and Stomach. The Liver Meridian is important to treat for any problems of the lower abdomen, for the Liver rules the lower "burning space" (see p. 118). It can therefore affect such diverse conditions as piles, constipation, and menstrual pain. Since the Liver belongs to the Wood element (see p. 100), you should also treat the Liver Meridian for muscular aches and cramps. Emotional stress, and repression (especially of anger) particularly affect the Liver; it is therefore involved in many of the conditions variously labelled in the West as "hysterical", or "psychosomatic". To the Oriental way of thinking, however, problems caused by emotional stress obstructing the *ki* of the Liver are as valid as any other. The Earth meridian of the Spleen is concerned with the digestive process and works with the kidneys to maintain the body's fluid balance. It also influences the menstrual cycle. The Stomach is another Earth meridian, chiefly concerned with the transformation of food into *ki* energy. On the Stomach Meridian one point in particular strengthens this function. Known as "Stomach 36" it is the best point for digestive problems, low energy and for increasing the body's resistance to disease.

Front of Leg Meridians
The Stomach and Spleen Meridians lie on each side of the big muscles at the front of the thigh. The Stomach Meridian runs down the outside, skirts the knee and goes down the outer edge of the shinbone. The Spleen Meridian lies along the inner edge of the thigh muscle, then joins the Liver Meridian on the inside of the shin.

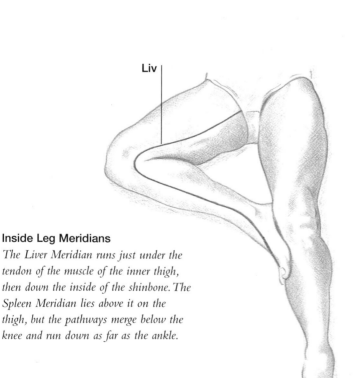

Inside Leg Meridians
The Liver Meridian runs just under the tendon of the muscle of the inner thigh, then down the inside of the shinbone. The Spleen Meridian lies above it on the thigh, but the pathways merge below the knee and run down as far as the ankle.

See Key to Meridians on p. 92

Front and Inside of Legs

When working on the front and inside of the legs, you are treating the meridians concerned with digestion, so the natural place for your "mother" hand is on the *hara*. It will often feel rumbles or gurgles as your other hand works down the meridians. To treat the Liver Meridian, you need to bend your partner's leg outward. And if the meridian is tight – as it is on almost everyone – you will have to support the leg at its point of maximum stretch, to avoid straining your partner's hip joint. The best way to support it is to lay the knee against your own thighs, as shown right. The points on the inside shin, just above the ankle, are often very tender, so try to work more gently on this area.

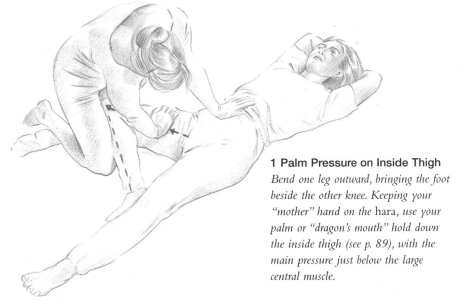

1 Palm Pressure on Inside Thigh

Bend one leg outward, bringing the foot beside the other knee. Keeping your "mother" hand on the hara, *use your palm or "dragon's mouth" hold down the inside thigh (see p. 89), with the main pressure just below the large central muscle.*

2 Heel of Hand Pressure down Inside Shin

Continuing down the leg, turn your hand as you pass the knee and use the heel of your hand to press gently down the groove beside the shinbone – the meridians run in that groove. Now straighten the leg again.

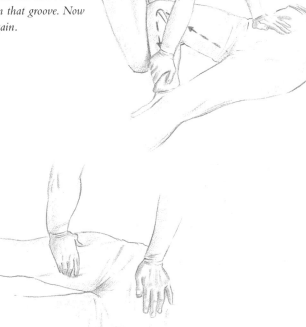

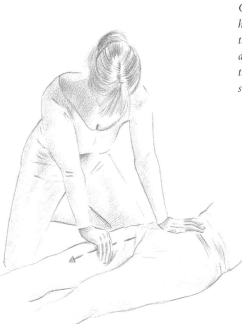

3 Palm Pressure on Front of Thigh

Press along both sides of the big muscle at the front of the thigh, grasping it at the same time, as shown right. Repeat once.

Front and Inside of Legs (II)

It is the Stomach and Spleen
Meridians that you are treating on the
front of the leg. Stomach 36, the
"wonder point" at the top of the shin,
dominates the sequence, as one of
the principal points for general well-
being. It may be a little hard to find at
first, but try finding it on yourself and
you will soon get a "feel" for where it is
on other people. So important is this
point that for once you can bring your
"mother" hand down from the *hara*
and use it to press Stomach 36
instead. If your partner's legs tend to
fall outward to the side, you may have
to support the leg you are working on
with your knee so that you can still
work with direct downward pressure.
When you have finished this sequence
on both legs, the shiatsu treatment is
complete. Cover your partner with a
blanket and allow him or her to rest for
a few minutes.

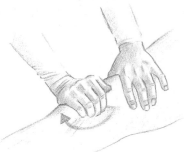

4 Rotating the Kneecap
*Still working on the same leg, use one
hand to support it near the knee and the
other to grasp the kneecap firmly and
rotate it two or three times in each
direction.*

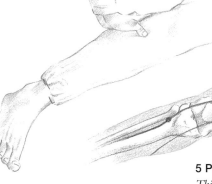

5 Pressing Stomach 36
*This point lies at the top of the shinbone,
in the curve where the bone widens
toward the knee, as shown above. To find
it, run your thumb up the outside of the
bone until you feel the curve. Then press
quite deeply and ask your partner how it
feels. If you are on the point, there should
be a strong sensation, which may run
down the meridian to the ankle. Once
you have located Stomach 36, bring your
"mother" hand down and hold the point
with your thumb.*

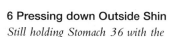

6 Pressing down Outside Shin
*Still holding Stomach 36 with the
thumb of your "mother" hand, use the
other thumb to press down the outside
of the shinbone. Repeat once.*

7 Stretching Foot Forward

Adopt a "racing start" position. Now holding the foot firmly, lift it off the ground and lean forward to stretch the leg.

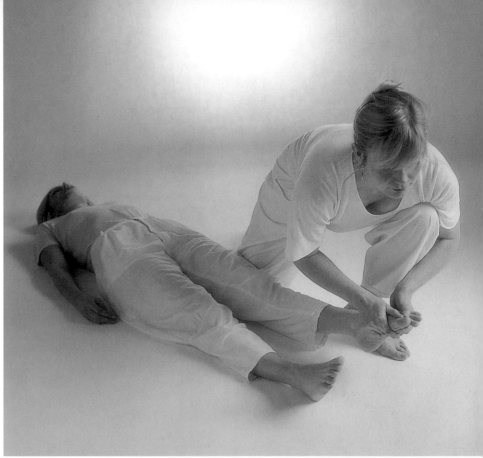

8 Stretching Foot Back

Still holding the foot, take your weight back on to your haunches and bring the foot back toward you. Repeat both movements once. Then move to the other side of your partner.

Repeat 1–8 on the other leg.

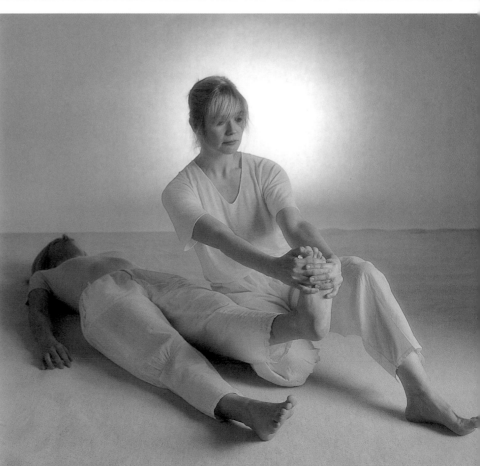

Shiatsu Checklist

This chart provides a quick checklist for you to use once you have learned the basic shiatsu techniques. You can consult it to remind you of the correct sequence for a full body treatment, while you are learning. A shiatsu massage should always be given over the whole body, to balance the energy in all the meridians. The sequence we present in this chapter is a basic routine aimed at relieving tension and promoting good health. Once you can do it without consulting the book, you may like to take a course in shiatsu and add new techniques to your repertoire (see p. 190).

Back of Body

Back *(pp. 92–5)*
1 Diagonal Stretch
2 Lumbar Stretch
3 Palm Pressure down Spine
4 Thumb Pressure down Spine

Hips *(pp. 96–9)*
1 Pressing the Sacral Holes
2 Squeezing the Hips
3 Elbow Pressure down Hips

**Back and Outside
of Legs** *(pp. 100–5)*
1 Palm Pressure on Back of Leg
2 Knee Pressure on Back of Leg
3 Pressing Ankle Tsubos
4 Three-Way Stretch
5 Palm Pressure down Side of Leg
6 Pressing Ankle Tsubo

Repeat 1–6 on the other leg

7 Walking on the Soles
8 Pressing Tsubo on Sole

9 Massaging the Heel
10 Pinching Outside of Foot
11 Pulling the Toes
12 Slapping the Sole
13 Pounding the Sole

Repeat 8–13 on the other foot

Back of Shoulders *(pp. 106–9)*
1 Thumb Pressure on Top of Shoulders
2 Elbowing between Blades
3 Rotating the Shoulderblades
4 Foot Pressure on Shoulders

Front of Body

**Front of Shoulders and
Neck** *(pp. 110–13)*
1 Leaning on the Shoulders
2 Pressing along the Ribs
3 Neck Sequence
4 Circling Sides of Neck
5 Stretching the Neck

Head and Face *(pp. 114–17)*
1 Running Hands through Hair
2 Pulling the Hair
3 Massaging the Ears
4 Pressing Top of Head Points
5 Eyes Sequence
6 Temples Sequence
7 Nose and Mouth Sequence

Arms and Hands *(pp. 118–21)*
1 Palm Pressure along Inner Arm
2 Grasping Upper Arm
3 Palm Pressure down Forearm
4 Pulling the Fingers
5 Pressing the "Great Eliminator"
6 Shaking the Arm

Repeat 1–6 on the other arm

Hara *(pp. 122–5)*
1 Lower Hara
2 Upper Hara
3 Rocking the Hara

Front and Inside of Legs *(pp. 126–9)*
1 Palm Pressure on Inside Thigh
*2 Heel of Hand Pressure down
   Inside Shin*
3 Palm Pressure on Front of Thigh
4 Rotating the Kneecap
5 Pressing Stomach 36
6 Pressing down Outside Shin
7 Stretching Foot Forward
8 Stretching Foot Back

Repeat 1–8 on the the other leg

Pressure Points for Massage

If you like the idea of shiatsu, but feel more at home with an oil massage, you may like to incorporate a few of the pressure points, or *tsubos*, into the Basic Massage Sequence given on pp. 36–7. Used within massage, these points will not have such a deep organic effect as in a shiatsu treatment, but they all stimulate the nervous system in specific ways and give a strong command to the muscles to relax.

Note: Most of these points are most easily reached with the thumb, although you may like to try your elbow on the points on the back. Press each point two or three times for about 3–5 seconds.

Back of Body

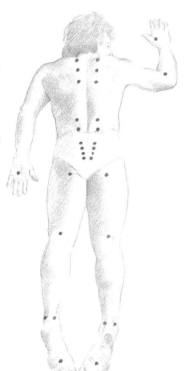

Back
● ● *each side of spine between vertebrae* → *balances all internal functions*

Hips
● ● *sides of buttocks (squeeze with heels of hands)* → *relaxes pelvis; unlocks* ki *to legs; relieves menstrual problems*
● ● *sacral holes* → *relieves pelvic congestion*
● *centre of buttock crease* → *relaxes muscles of lower back and hips*

Legs
● *back of knee (support the knee and dig fairly deeply with both thumbs)* → *relieves sciatica*

Ankles
● *both sides of Achilles tendon at once* → *stimulates Water functions; relieves low back pain*

Feet
● *under centre of ball of foot* → *calms and relaxes*

Key
● = *location of point*
→ = *effect*

Front of Body

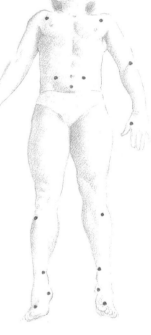

Head and Face
(see pp. 114, 116 and 117 for head and face points)

Shoulders
● *about 4 cm (1½ inches) below hollow at outer end of collarbone* → *stimulates lung function*

Arms and Hands
● *"Great Eliminator" (p. 121) (pinch)* → *eliminates colds, headaches and toothache*
● *centre of palm* → *calms mind and emotions*
● *outside of elbow at outside end of crease when arm is bent* → *tonifies Large Intestine and relieves arm and shoulder pain*

Hara
● ● *about 7 cm (3 inches) either side of navel (press in toward navel)* → *stimulates intestines and relaxes stomach tension*
● *Tan-Den (p. 122) (press deeply with flat of four fingers)* → *stimulates whole body*

Legs
● *Stomach 36 (p. 128)* → *promotes general energy and well-being*
● *four fingers up from inner ankle bone next to shin* → *calms; relieves period pains*

Feet
● *about 2.5 to 5 cm (1–2 inches) above join between big toe and second toe* → *harmonizes Liver energy*
● *centre of inside heel* → *stimulates Kidney function*

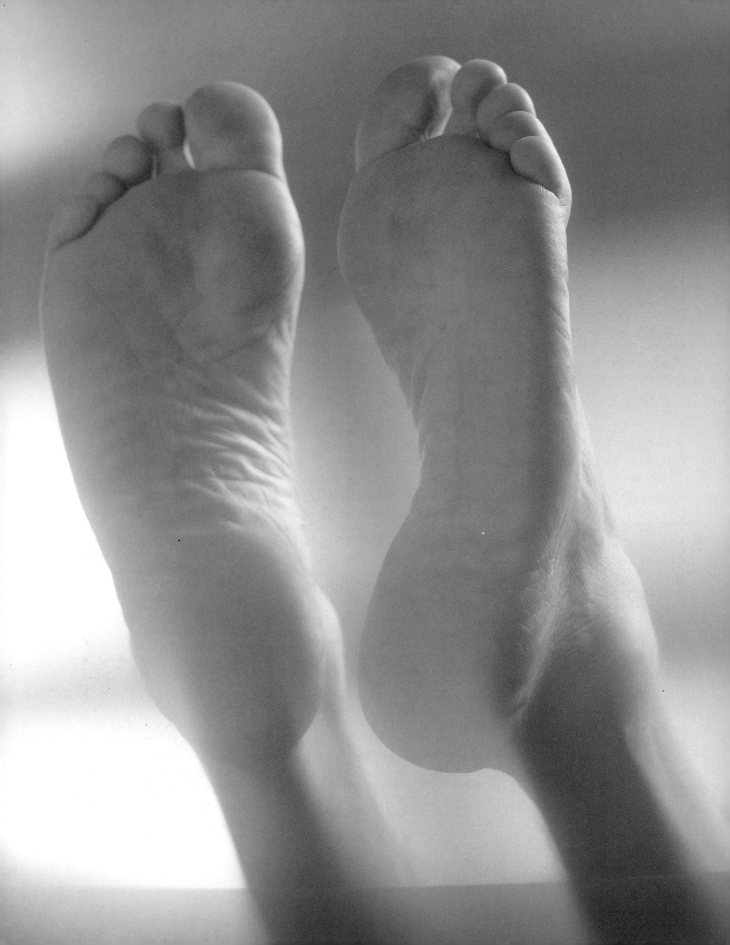

Reflexology

Reflexology is based on the principle that there are areas, or reflex points, on the feet and hands that correspond to each organ, gland and structure in the body. By working on these reflexes, the reflexologist reduces tension all over the body.

The precise origins of reflexology are not known, but it may well have originated around the same time as acupuncture – about 4000 BC – for the two share many of the same principles. And it was certainly in use in Egypt about 2330 BC, as shown by the detail from the wall painting on page 13. Its modern origins, however, are easier to trace. In 1917, an American physician, Dr William H. Fitzgerald, laid the foundations of the science with his "zone therapy". This postulated the existence of ten zones of energy, dividing the body from head to feet. By applying pressure to certain parts of the fingers with his hands and various mechanical devices, Dr Fitzgerald discovered that he could relieve pain in other parts of the body in the same zone. But the science was established in its present form mainly through an American therapist called Eunice Ingham, encouraged initially by Dr J.S. Riley, the physician for whom she was working. She discovered that the feet were more responsive to pressure than the hands and instated them as the major area of treatment. From the early 1930s until her death in 1974, Eunice Ingham worked ceaselessly to develop reflexology into the science it is today. The International Institute of Reflexology was founded in 1973 to carry on her work.

No one knows exactly how reflexology works, although several theories exist. The Institute adheres to the view that energy is constantly flowing through channels or zones in the body that terminate to form the reflex points on the feet and hands. When this energy flow is unimpeded, we remain healthy, but when it is blocked by tension or congestion, disease occurs. Through treating the reflexes, the blocks are broken down and harmony is restored to all systems.

A typical reflexology treatment lasts about 30–40 minutes. Taking one foot at a time, you work on the reflexes on the sole, side and top, using the appropriate thumb and finger techniques. Skill as a reflexologist depends largely on experience – it takes time and practice to detect the reflexes that are tender and develop the sensitivity in your fingers to treat them. After working over a painful reflex a few times, you leave it to treat another one, then return to concentrate on it once again until the pain is no longer acute. It may take several sessions, however, until the tenderness disappears completely. In your eagerness to get rid of the pain, don't overwork a reflex.

The main benefit of reflexology is relaxation. But in reducing tension you also improve the blood supply, bring about unimpeded nerve functioning and re-establish harmony or homeostasis among all body functions. Since most of today's diseases stem from the effects of stress, a reflexology treatment from a qualified practitioner can be of enormous benefit for a wide range of conditions.

As a student of reflexology, however, it is not your prerogative to diagnose or treat medical problems. If you are in doubt about any medical conditions, always consult a doctor before treating someone. And be sure to observe any contraindications given in this chapter. Your aim should be to relax and tone up your partner. Reflexology is an intricate and exact science. This chapter is simply designed as an introduction to some of the basic techniques. If you seriously want to practise it professionally, you should attend the special teaching seminars run by the Institute (see p. 190).

Theory and Principles

As a beginner to reflexology, it is important to study the principles on which the science is based – particularly the zone theory (below) and the reflexes charts (pp. 136–7 and 148–9). These constitute the grammar of reflexology, enabling you to understand how you can relax different parts of the body by treating specific reflexes. The zone theory (below) subdivides the body into ten zones, each running through the length of the body. It will help you to familiarize yourself with the theory if you mentally travel up the body from each toe, visualizing the parts of your own body which lie within each zone. The foot guidelines (opposite) enable you to apply the reflexes charts to any shape or size of foot, showing you how to orientate yourself with each new partner.

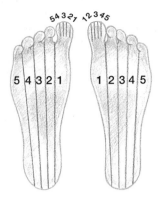

The Zones on the Feet
Each of your toes represents a zone which travels the length of the body. All the toes are reflex areas for the head, but the major reflexes for the head are in the big toes. Each big toe represents half the head and each therefore subdivides into five zones.

The Zone Theory

The zone theory explains the link between the reflexes on the feet and the parts of the body to which they correspond. According to this theory there are ten "zones" or energy channels running longitudinally up the body from feet to head – five on each side, one for each finger or toe, as shown right. Any organ, gland or part of the body that is situated within a certain zone will have its reflex in the corresponding zone of the foot (or hand). Thus the reflex for the spine runs along the inside of both feet (Zone 1), and the reflex for the liver across the outer four zones of the right foot (Zones 2, 3, 4, 5). Overlaying the zone lines on an anatomical figure, as far right, makes it easier to visualize how treating a reflex point in any one zone of the foot will affect any part of the body within the same zone. If you come across a tender area while treating the foot, it often means there is tension or congestion in the part of the body which lies in the same zone. In fact, any condition that interferes with the flow of energy at any point along one of the zones will have a detrimental effect on all structures that share that zone.

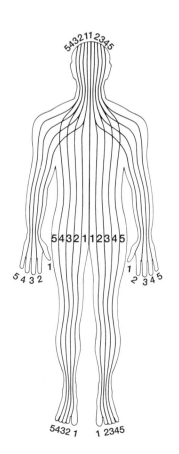

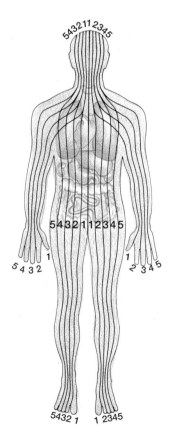

The Bones of the Foot

If you are to practise as a reflexologist, you should acquire a working knowledge of the bones of the foot – for it is partly from these that you orientate yourself before beginning a treatment. Each foot consists of 26 bones – 7 tarsal bones, 5 metatarsals (the long bones in the middle), and the 14 phalanges of the toes. Explore your own feet with your hands and try to feel how the bones are arranged.

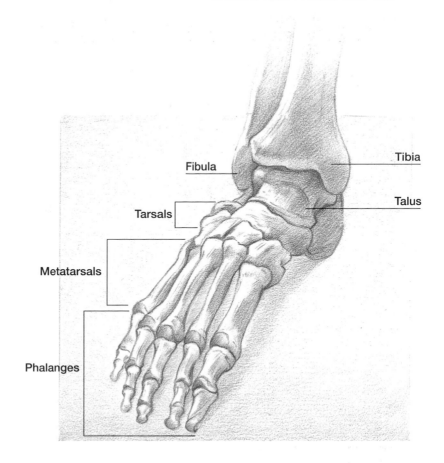

Guidelines on the Feet

You cannot work on an unfamiliar pair of feet simply by referring to the chart of foot reflexes. Feet, like people, come in all different shapes and sizes. To find your bearings on each individual pair of feet, you first need to locate certain "landmarks" or guidelines. There are three guidelines running laterally across the feet – the Diaphragm Line, the Waist Line, and the Heel Line. These allow you to orientate yourself so that you can then home in on the reflexes accurately. The Diaphragm Line runs across the feet just below the ball of the foot, the heads of the metatarsals. The Waist Line can be found by drawing an imaginary line across the foot from the protrusion on the outside of the foot, the fifth metatarsal. To locate the Heel Line, look for the point just above the heel, where the lighter, softer skin of the arch area changes into the darker, thicker skin of the heel. Once you have located these three guidelines you will be able to determine the exact position of the reflexes that lie above or below them.

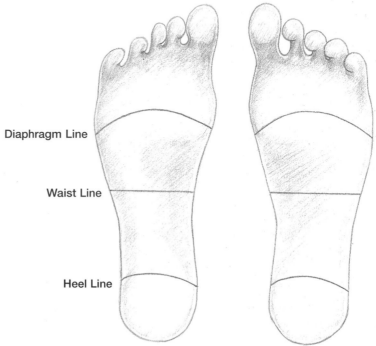

Foot Reflexes Chart

This chart shows the exact location of the reflexes of various parts of the body on the soles and outsides of the feet. As you can see, the reflexes on the two soles are very similar; some, however, appear on one foot only, because the organs to which they correspond lie on one side of the body – the heart, for example, is on the left sole, the liver on the right. For the sake of simplicity, only some reflexes are represented here – although, in fact, every single organ, gland, and structure of the body has a reflex on the feet. We have reproduced the feet on these pages exactly as they look when you are treating someone – that is, their right sole faces your left hand, their left sole your right hand. Experienced reflexologists see themselves dealing directly with various structures within the body, rather than just working on the feet.

The Foot/Body Relationship

The foot reflexes represent a remarkably accurate map of the body, mirroring the location of the various parts, as shown below. Notice how the Diaphragm Reflex matches the diaphragm on the anatomy, for example. If you imagine the two feet moving together to cover the torso you will see how the Spinal Reflexes fall along the inside edge of both feet.

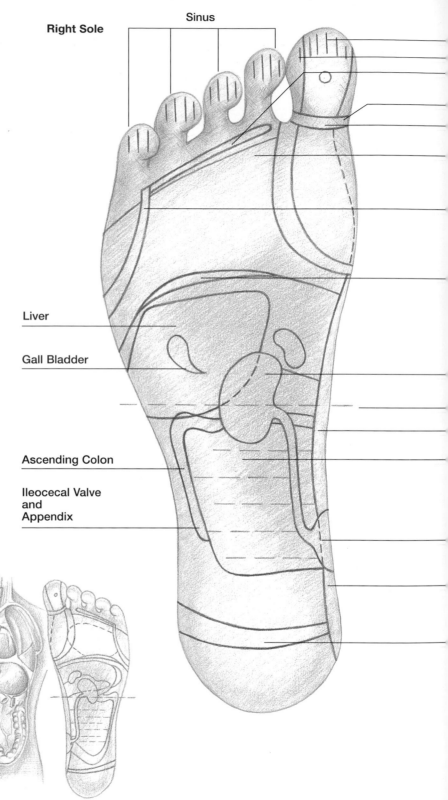

Right Sole

Sinus

Liver

Gall Bladder

Ascending Colon

Ileocecal Valve and Appendix

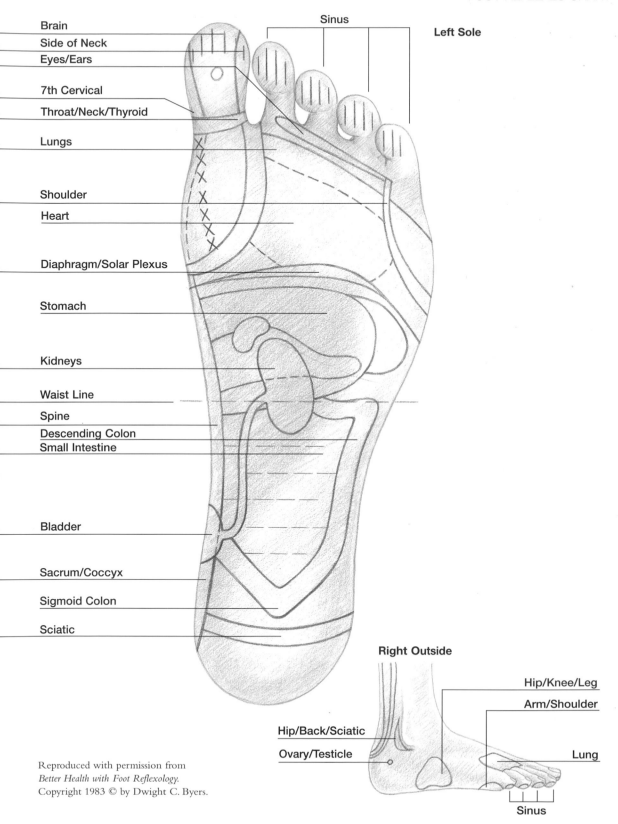

Brain
Side of Neck
Eyes/Ears

7th Cervical
Throat/Neck/Thyroid

Lungs

Shoulder

Heart

Diaphragm/Solar Plexus

Stomach

Kidneys

Waist Line

Spine
Descending Colon
Small Intestine

Bladder

Sacrum/Coccyx

Sigmoid Colon

Sciatic

Sinus

Left Sole

Right Outside

Hip/Knee/Leg

Arm/Shoulder

Lung

Hip/Back/Sciatic

Ovary/Testicle

Sinus

Reproduced with permission from
Better Health with Foot Reflexology.
Copyright 1983 © by Dwight C. Byers.

Basic Techniques

The finger and thumb techniques of reflexology are unlike any other strokes or movements used in the natural healing arts, and will take some time to master. Ideally, you should try to attend a seminar or course while learning, but if this is not possible, study these basic techniques closely and spend some time practising them before attempting the treatment sequence. In addition to the relaxation techniques featured opposite, there are four basic working techniques – thumb, index finger, hooking, and reflex rotation. Most reflexology treatment is done with the basic thumb and index finger techniques, moving forward like a caterpillar across each reflex, using both hands. Hooking and reflex rotation are more specialized techniques, used on certain reflexes only.

Caution: *Do not treat people with varicose veins, unless you use the referral areas (see p. 163). And, apart from the gentle relaxation techniques, avoid practising reflexology on pregnant women, unless you are properly qualified.*

Practical Matters

The beauty of reflexology is that you can give it anywhere, at any time – all you really need is your hands. The only proviso is that both you and the receiver should be as comfortable as possible. The receiver's feet should be at about the same level as your lap, so that you don't need to bend over too far. Apart from a couple of chairs, all that is necessary is a little talcum powder or cornflour to put on if the receiver's feet are damp, and a towel to cover your lap. (Oils or creams are never used in reflexology.) And you should make sure that your nails are short before a session.

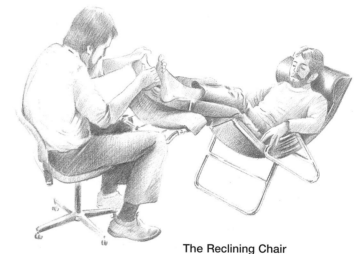

The Reclining Chair
This provides the ideal position for someone receiving reflexology, giving firm support for head and knees and allowing complete relaxation.

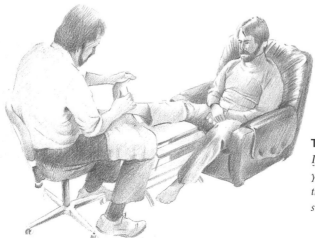

The Armchair and Stool
If you don't possess a reclining chair, seat your partner on an armchair or sofa with the leg you are working on supported on a stool of similar height.

Relaxation Techniques

Relaxation is the key to effective reflexology. At the start of a treatment, you
use the three techniques shown here,
first on one foot and then the other, to
accustom the receiver to your hands
and relax the feet. You should also
return to them to soothe the receiver
after working any painful reflexes in the
course of treatment, and after
completing the full treatment sequence
on each foot. Of the three techniques
presented here, always use Back and
Forth first, following it with either of the
other two techniques. The Diaphragm
and Solar Plexus Flexing technique is
particularly beneficial for people who
suffer from tension.

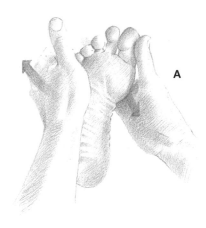

Back and Forth

*Place the palms of your hands on either
side of the foot, fingers relaxed (A).
Now gently push forward with one hand
and pull back with the other (B).
Continue this movement, alternately
pushing and pulling the foot back and
forth fairly rapidly, keeping your hands
constantly in contact with the foot.*

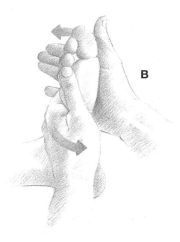

Diaphragm and Solar Plexus Flexing

A *Press your thumb firmly into the arch
just below the ball of the foot (the
Diaphragm and Solar Plexus Reflex),
right thumb on right foot, and left hand
supporting. Grasp the base of the toes
with the supporting hand.*

B *Now gently flex the toes toward you,
pulling the foot against the thumb.
Beginning at the inside edge of the reflex,
slowly inch your thumb across toward the
outside edge.*

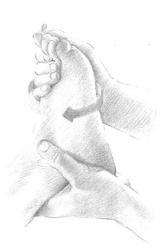

Ankle Rotation

*Support the heel in the opposite hand –
right heel in left hand and vice versa –
with your thumb around the outside of
the ankle, just below the ankle bone. Now
grasp the top of the foot in your other
hand and gently rotate it a few times in
one direction, then a few in the other.*

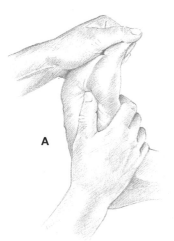

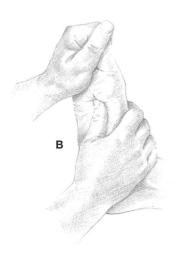

Basic Holding Technique

To be a good reflexologist, you need to develop teamwork between your hands – one hand holds the foot steady while the other hand works the reflexes. Each of the various working techniques entails a slightly different hold – a variation on the basic holding technique shown right. You always use both hands on each foot, so be sure to practise this basic handhold both ways around, until it feels natural.

Basic Holding Technique

To work on the right foot, wrap your left hand around the toes, holding them straight without bending them forward or back excessively, and use your right hand for working. Now change hands. To work on the left foot, start by using your right hand as the "holding" hand and then change over.

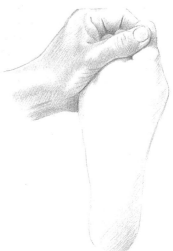

Basic Thumb Technique

In reflexology you use your thumbs mainly to work the reflexes on the soles, and sometimes the sides, of the feet. Working with the first joint of your thumb you "walk" forward along the reflex by successively bending and unbending the joint a little way. It is the inside or medial edge of the thumb that makes contact with the foot, not the tip or the ball (the part that touches the table if you put your hand down flat).

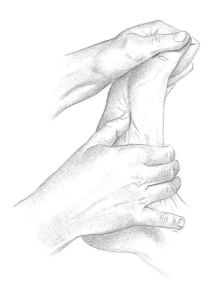

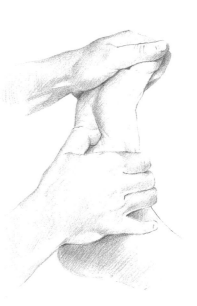

Basic Thumb Technique

When the thumb is at the correct angle, the joint is not bent too far, allowing greater accuracy and smoothness of technique, as shown above. Bending the joint over too far, as shown right, not only strains it but also means that the person you are working on may feel your nail. The fingers of the "working" hand wrap around the top of the foot to provide leverage.

Index Finger Technique

The index finger comes into play when you are working on the top and side of the foot. Once again, you make contact with the inside or medial edge of the finger, bending the joint slightly to "walk" or creep forward. This time, the thumb gives leverage from the other side of the foot and pushes the metatarsal head forward, to make working the top of the foot easier. Practise the movement until you can execute it smoothly, keeping the pressure steady. Try "walking" over a painful reflex in one direction with your left index finger, then come back over it with your right.

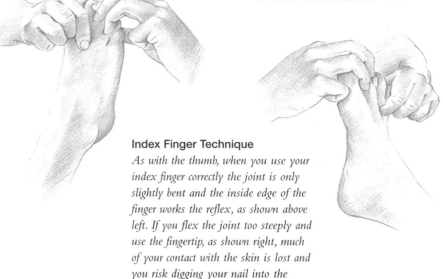

Index Finger Technique
As with the thumb, when you use your index finger correctly the joint is only slightly bent and the inside edge of the finger works the reflex, as shown above left. If you flex the joint too steeply and use the fingertip, as shown right, much of your contact with the skin is lost and you risk digging your nail into the person receiving treatment.

Hooking

This technique is useful for homing in on a particularly small reflex and for working on parts of the foot where the skin is tough, such as the heel. Like a bee inserting a sting, you push your thumb into the reflex, then pull it back. The leverage of the fingers is crucial here, as the technique demands great precision.

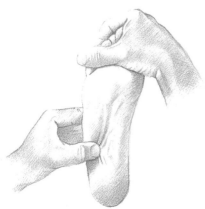

Hooking
Support the foot well in your "holding" hand and place the thumb of your "working" hand on a reflex area. Now hook the thumb in and back up sharply, to one side (in this instance, toward the outside).

Reflex Rotation

Specifically designed to help "work out" a painful reflex, this technique is used on the reflexes to the upper abdominal area of both feet, (that is, between the Waist Line and Diaphragm Line). You should apply it if you come across a particularly tender area, keeping your thumb in position while you rotate the foot around it, as shown below. After a few minutes of the reflex rotation, you will find that the pain has diminished considerably. Go gently, being careful to avoid digging your thumbnail in.

Reflex Rotation
Press your "working" thumb gently onto the reflex. Now use the "holding" hand to rotate the upper foot around the thumb, clockwise then anticlockwise.

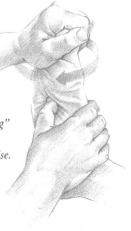

Foot Treatment Sequence

When treating a pair of feet for the first time, begin by checking for any hard skin, calluses, corns, and so on that might interfere with the flow of energy in that zone. If you discover any problems, advise your friend to seek treatment from a chiropodist. Now orientate yourself with the feet, as shown on page 135. After thoroughly relaxing both feet, you will begin to work on the reflexes, completing the whole sequence on one foot, then repeating it on the other. The sequence proceeds systematically down the foot, from toes to heel – from the head to the lower abdominal reflexes – then up the inside edge of the foot to work on the spinal reflexes. When initially learning the sequence, each time you come to a new reflex zone, study the foot reflexes chart (see pp. 136–7) and note the exact position of the reflexes. During the treatment, give more attention to any painful areas you discover and after working both feet return briefly to rework these areas, one foot at a time. But don't expect to get rid of them in one session. Always go gently – overworking sensitive points is counter-productive, creating tension rather than relaxation.

The Head, Sinus, Eye, and Ear Reflexes

All the toes contain reflexes to the head, those on the right foot to the right side of the head, and vice versa. The main reflexes are found on the big toes; the smaller toes are the "fine tune" reflexes for the head, as well as the sinuses. If someone has a bad tooth, say, you will find their toe in the corresponding zone sensitive. If the sinuses are congested, all the toes will be painful to the touch. Working the toes takes a lot of practice – not only are they sensitive, but their size makes them difficult to hold and treat. You treat the Eye and Ear Reflexes most directly at the base of the smaller toes. Since it is tension that is at the root of many eye problems, preventing proper circulation and focusing, reflexology is often very effective, restoring normal functioning by promoting relaxation.

Head and Sinus Reflexes

To treat the left foot, support and protect the toes with the right hand and use your left thumb to work on the reflexes, keeping your left fingers over your right. Starting at the big toe, let your thumb "walk" down to the base of each toe in a small "caterpillar" movement. When you reach the little toe, change hands and "walk" back toward the big toe again. Reverse the instructions for the right foot.

Eye and Ear Reflexes

To treat these reflex areas, you "walk" along the ridge at the base of the little toes formed by the metatarsal joints. With one hand, support the foot and use the thumb to pull down the fleshy skin covering the base of the toes. Use the outside edge of both thumbs to "walk" along the ridge in both directions.

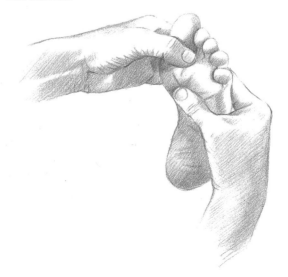

The Neck and Throat Reflex

The reflex zone for the neck and throat lies at the base of the big toe. Working with this zone affects not only the neck itself but also the top of the spine, the tonsils and the thyroid and parathyroid glands.

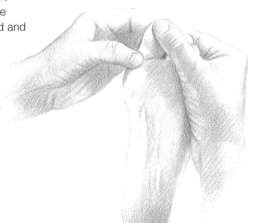

Neck and Throat Reflex

Supporting the foot with one hand, use the other thumb to work around the base of the big toe from the side, then change hands and come back in the opposite direction, reversing which hand holds and which thumb works the reflex.

The Lung Reflex

This reflex area is situated between the metatarsal joints and the base of the toes on the sole of the foot, and between the metatarsal bones on the top of the foot. You begin by working on the Lung Reflex area on the sole of the foot, as shown right, then treat the top of the foot. The Lung Reflex areas affect all the organs within the thoracic cavity, not just the lungs.

Lung Reflex on Sole

Hold the toes in one hand, and use the medial corner of the other thumb to work up between the metatarsals to the base of the toes. Then work back in the opposite direction using the other thumb.

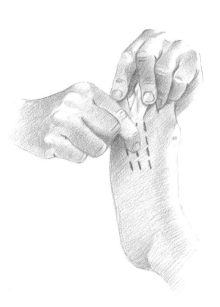

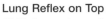

Lung Reflex on Top

Hold the toes in one hand and use the medial, or inside, corner of your other index finger to work down between the metatarsal bones from the base of each toe. Start at the big toe and work across to the little toe. Then change hands and work back the other way. Your thumbs should push forward on the heads of the metatarsals to open up the top of the foot.

The Upper Abdominal Area

This large reflex zone lies between the Waist Line and the heads of the metatarsal joints (Diaphragm Line). Since the reflexes to organs on the right-hand side of the body are located on the right foot and vice versa, you will find the Liver Reflex mainly on the right foot and the Stomach and Pancreas Reflexes mainly on the left. The Kidney Reflexes are on both feet. Our foot treatment sequence concentrates only on the Liver. If either foot is particularly painful to the touch in the upper abdominal area, use reflex rotation (see p. 141) in addition to the basic thumb technique.

Liver Reflex

With your "holding" hand on the toes, work systematically across the whole area with your thumb. Be sure to wrap the fingers of your "working" hand around the top of the foot to give leverage to the thumb. Once again, use alternate hands as the "working" hand.

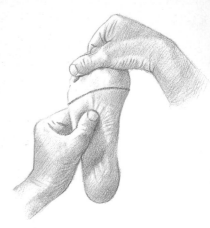

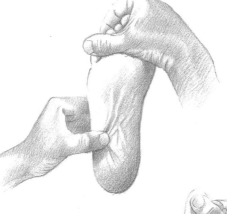

Ileocecal Valve, Appendix, and Ascending Colon Reflexes

Place your left thumb on the Ileocecal Valve and Appendix Reflex and hook back toward the outside of the foot, using the hooking technique (p. 141). Now "walk" your thumb up the outside of the foot until the Waist Line, to work the entire Ascending Colon Reflex area.

The Lower Abdominal Area

The reflexes to the ascending colon and the ileocecal valve are on the right foot. To find the Ileocecal Valve and Appendix Reflex, "walk" your left thumb slowly up the inside edge of the foot until you find a tender point, just above the heel bone. The Ascending Colon Reflex continues up from this point to the level of the Waist Line. As well as digestive disorders, bronchial problems, asthma and allergic conditions also respond well to treatment of this area. Working the Sigmoid and Descending Colon Reflexes helps flatulence, constipation and other stress-related conditions. Both reflexes are on the left foot. The Sigmoid Colon Reflex on the heel bone is difficult to work with because the skin is very tough here. The Descending Colon Reflex runs up the outside edge of the foot to the Waist Line, as shown right. This area is often tender, due to lack of exercise, stress, and a deficiency in dietary fibre.

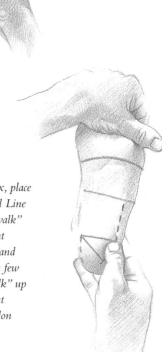

Sigmoid and Descending Colon Reflexes

To locate the Sigmoid Colon Reflex, place your left thumb just above the Heel Line on the inside of the left foot and "walk" down at a 45° angle until the point marked, as above. Now hook back and forth toward the inside of the foot a few times. Then change hands and "walk" up the outside of the foot with the right thumb to work the Descending Colon Reflex area, as shown right.

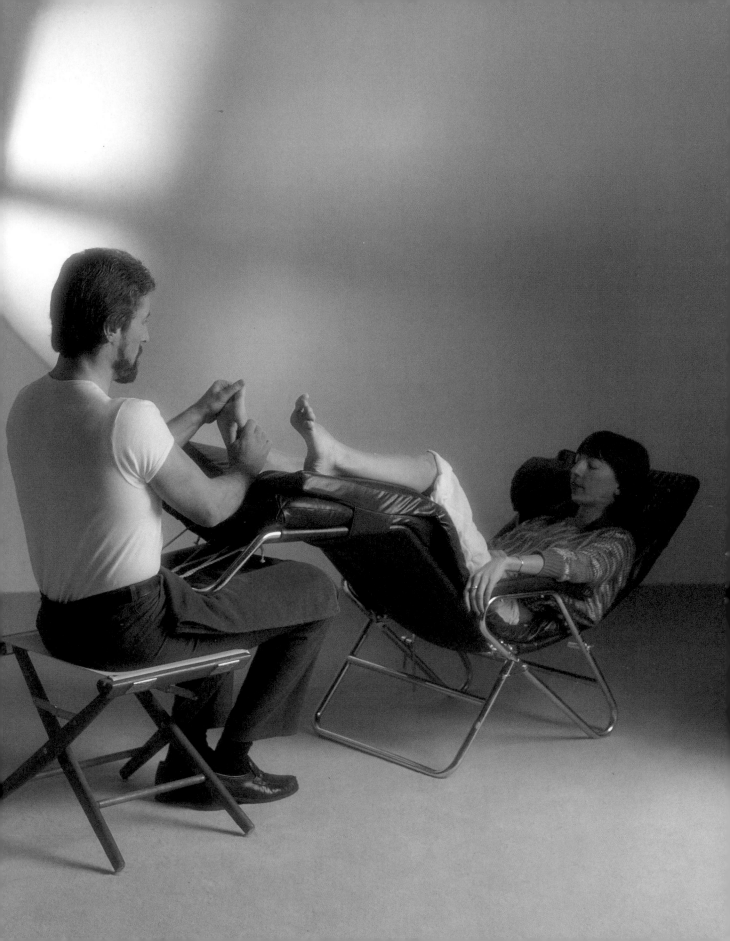

The Spinal Reflexes

You work the Spinal Reflexes in one continuous motion along the inside edge of each foot – from the coccyx and sacrum area which begins at the inside edge of each heel. This is one of the most important of all reflexes, for the health of the spine is central to the well-being of the whole body. Stress, poor posture and lack of exercise can create tension and imbalance in the network of muscles supporting the spine, and this in turn not only causes backache but also impedes the functioning of the spinal nerves which link the brain with the rest of the body. Since relaxation is the primary effect of reflexology, treating the Spinal Reflexes can have a most beneficial effect.

The Spine/Foot Relationship

There is an extraordinary similarity between the shape of the spine and the shape of its reflex on the inside of the foot, as shown right. Both have 26 bones and the four arches of the feet mirror the four curves of the spine – cervical, thoracic, lumbar, and sacral.

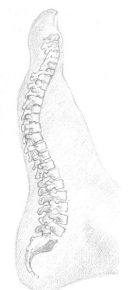

Cervical Area

Thoracic Area

Lumbar Area

Coccyx/ Sacrum Area

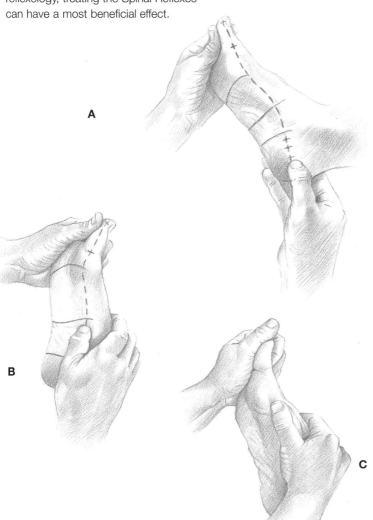

A

B

C

The Spinal Reflexes

To work the Spinal Reflexes (A) you start at the inside edge of the heel and "walk" your thumb up gradually toward the big toe. At the coccyx and sacrum area of the reflex the skin is generally rather tough, requiring you to exert more pressure than usual. This means wrapping the fingers of your "working" hand around the outside of the heel bone to give leverage to your "working" thumb. Work up the Spinal Reflexes as far as you can go without overstretching the thumb, then move the fingers of the working hand from the outside of the heel and place them over the instep as shown (B). With your "working" hand in this position, you will easily be able to continue up the lumbar, thoracic, and cervical areas of the reflex (C). If you discover any particularly tender spots, give them extra attention by "walking" over them a few times.

The Lower Back and Leg Area

Working the two reflex areas shown on this page is essential for all cases of backache, as well as for hip, knee, and leg problems. The reflexes are so-called "helper" areas – not only do they relax those parts of the body to which they directly correspond, but they also help to alleviate lower back pain. The Hip/Knee/Leg Reflex is a fairly large area on the outside of the foot, extending from the fifth metatarsal to the heel. If the person you are working on has a knee problem, the corresponding reflex on the same side will be very sensitive. The Hip/Back/Sciatic Reflex runs around the back of the ankle joint (see p. 137). Pain in this reflex often indicates sciatica.

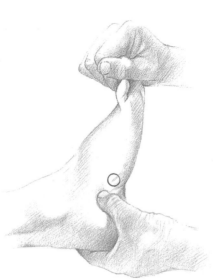

The Hip/Knee/Leg Reflex

You can work this area either with your index finger, as shown below, or with your thumb, as shown left. "Walk" across it in various directions, making a mental note of the difference between the two feet.

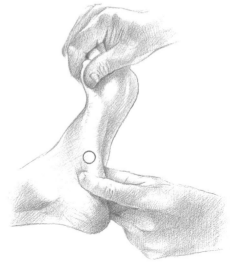

The Hip/Back/Sciatic Reflex

Hold the foot upright with your supporting hand. (If you allow the foot to tip forward the tendons will tighten, preventing you from working the reflex properly.) Now use your index finger to work thoroughly around the ankle joint.

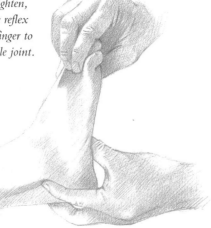

Hand Reflexes Chart

The positions of the hand reflexes correspond to those on the feet. But just as the hands and feet differ in shape and size, so too do their reflexes – the Spinal Reflexes are shorter on the hands, for example, and the Sinus Reflexes larger because the fingers are longer than the toes. The hand reflexes lie far deeper than those on the feet, since the hands are more exposed and so less sensitive. This makes them much harder to treat because it is more difficult to locate the tender spots.

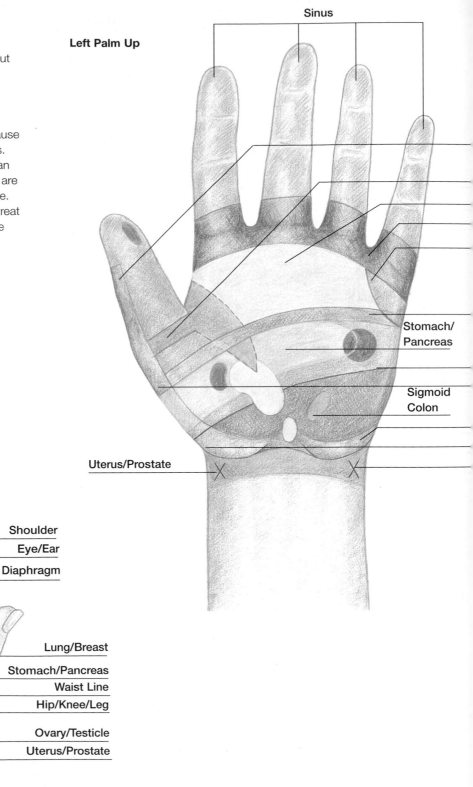

Left Palm Up

Sinus

Stomach/Pancreas

Sigmoid Colon

Uterus/Prostate

Sinus

Shoulder

Eye/Ear

Diaphragm

Lung/Breast

Stomach/Pancreas

Waist Line

Hip/Knee/Leg

Ovary/Testicle

Uterus/Prostate

Left Palm Down

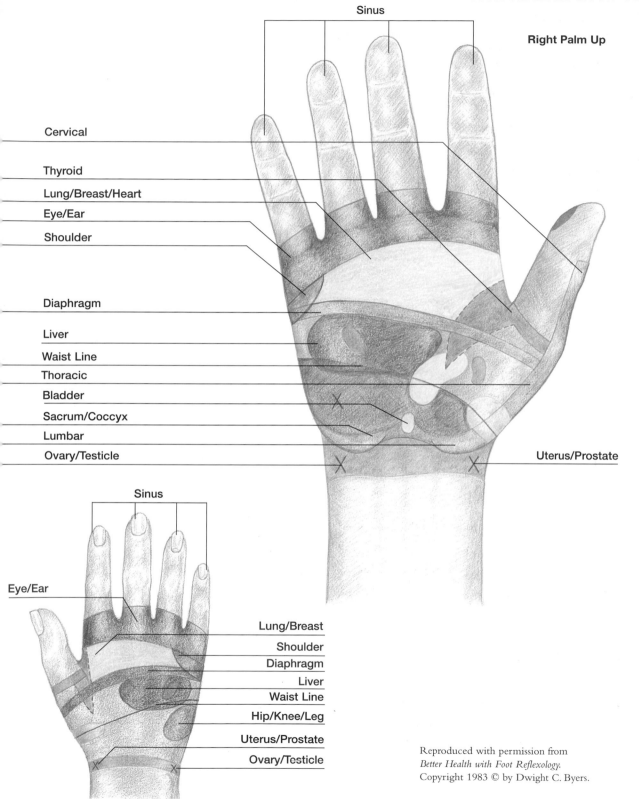

Sinus

Right Palm Up

Cervical

Thyroid

Lung/Breast/Heart

Eye/Ear

Shoulder

Diaphragm

Liver

Waist Line

Thoracic

Bladder

Sacrum/Coccyx

Lumbar

Ovary/Testicle

Uterus/Prostate

Sinus

Eye/Ear

Lung/Breast

Shoulder

Diaphragm

Liver

Waist Line

Hip/Knee/Leg

Uterus/Prostate

Ovary/Testicle

Right Palm Down

Reproduced with permission from
Better Health with Foot Reflexology.
Copyright 1983 © by Dwight C. Byers.

Hand Treatment Sequence

The main advantage of working on the hands rather than the feet is convenience – you can work on yourself or a partner anywhere, without needing to take anything off. But in general it is a less effective form of treatment because the reflexes are deeper and more difficult to contact. When treating the hands, you use your thumbs to work the palm and your index fingers to work the grooves between the fingers on the backs of the hands. The basic thumb technique is the same as for the feet – the only difference is that you continually extend and flex the hand onto your thumb as it "walks" forward.

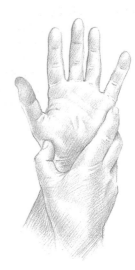

Diaphragm Relaxation

To find the Diaphragm Reflex, first locate the slight protuberance formed by the head of the fifth metacarpal bone – beneath the little finger – and the protuberance under the head of the first – at the base of the thumb. The reflex lies across both sides of the hand, just beneath these two protuberances, As well as being a vital part of our respiratory system, the diaphragm is also a frequent repository of tension and stress. It is thus a key reflex for relaxing the whole body. The relaxation technique used is virtually the same as the "Diaphragm Flexing" on the feet (see p.139).

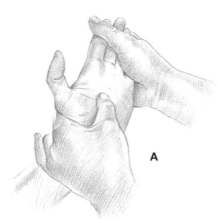

A

Diaphragm Relaxation Technique
Holding the hand firmly in one of your hands, place your other thumb on the middle of the Diaphragm Reflex (A). Now, as you "walk" the thumb gradually across the reflex, keep flexing the hand on to the thumb (B). Repeat on the other hand.

Self-help on the Spine
If you suffer from backache you can often relieve it yourself by working on the Spinal Reflexes with your thumb, supporting the fingers of your "working" hand, as shown above. The Lumbar Reflex area in particular is generally painful if you have a low back problem. Gently work on this area for a few minutes each day.

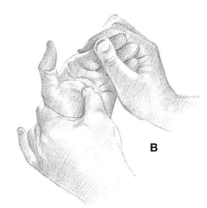

B

The Lung Reflex

This reflex is just above the Diaphragm Line on the back and palm of each hand. You treat it with your thumb on the palm, and then with your index finger on the back of the hand, using the same technique for both.

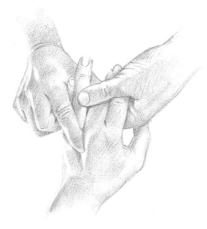

The Lung Reflex
Hold your partner's hand, as for the Diaphragm Relaxation. Now work down between the metacarpal bones with your thumb, while gently flexing and extending the fingers with your "holding" hand. Repeat on the back of the hand, as shown left.

The Liver Reflex

Below the Diaphragm Line on the right hand, you will find the Liver Reflex. Although this reflex is discernible on both sides of the hand, it is sometimes easier to detect on the back of the hand.

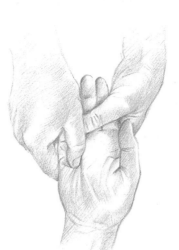

The Liver Reflex

"Walk" your thumb gradually across the reflex, while extending and flexing the hand gently against it, as shown left and right.

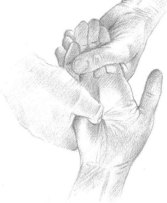

The Spinal Reflexes

Unlike most of the reflexes on the hand, the Spinal Reflexes are relatively easy to find and are very useful for self-help, as shown opposite, or for treating others. Before working the reflex, study the hand reflexes chart on pages 148–9, noting the different location of these reflexes here and on the feet.

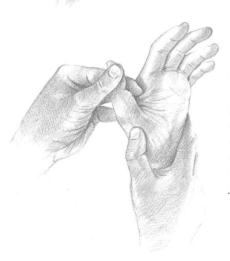

Spinal Reflexes

Starting at the heel of the hand, "walk" your thumb along the reflex from the lower back to the cervical area, using the same "caterpillar" motion as on the feet. Since the skin covering the reflexes is comparatively thin, it is not necessary to flex the hand.

The Hip/Knee/Leg Reflex

As on the feet, this reflex is a "helper" area for the spine, and can be effectively worked for all cases of backache. You will find it on the back of each hand, near the outside edge below the Waist Line. If it is tender, work the pain out gradually over several treatments.

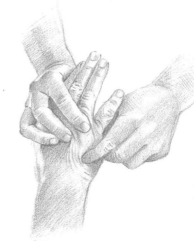

Hip/Knee/Leg Reflex

Use your index finger to "walk" gently over the whole area — first with one hand as the "working" hand, then with the other.

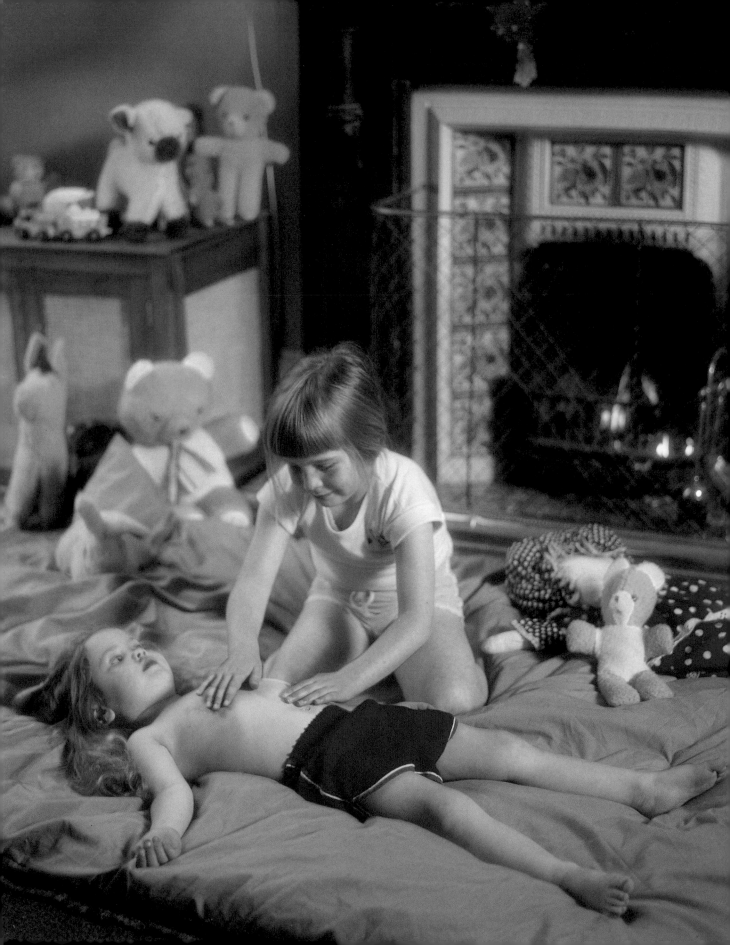

The Human Touch

Whatever our age or stage in life, we all need a little of the human touch, of the tenderness and caring that show us we are not alone. We are sentient beings – without the warmth of touch to link and soothe us, we are denied one of our most vital ways of communicating, of giving and receiving.

Some people think of massage as a luxury, and turn to it only at times of dire need. But given the pressures of modern society, and particularly the increase in stress-related illnesses, the touch therapies should become an integral part of everyday life, and should be recognized as a valuable ingredient of preventive health – both for the practitioner and the receiver. There is no doubt that giving any form of massage is almost as therapeutic as receiving it. Apart from the obvious satisfaction of helping people, treating someone with massage, shiatsu or reflexology can also relax you and enable you to cope with your own tension.

According to Oriental medicine, there are certain times in life, called "Gateways of Change", where you can actually improve your basic constitution if you take proper care of yourself – and permanently damage your health if you neglect yourself. These times are puberty, marriage (or the onset of sexual activity), pregnancy, childbirth and just after, and the menopause. During these periods, in particular, the touch therapies can be of enormous benefit, helping to provide the necessary relaxation to deal with hormonal change. In fact it is at times of stress that our need for physical contact is most intense, that we yearn for the release of tension it brings and the reassurance that our troubles are shared.

The three touch techniques taught in this book are suitable for everyone, but you will need to modify your treatment slightly for certain ages and circumstances of life. In this chapter we look at some of these special applications – Maternity, Babies, Later Life, Massage and Exercise, and Self-massage. Much of the advice given here is common sense – for instance you should naturally work more gently with babies and old people and make sure that the room you are working in is very warm. How you use the techniques you have learned will depend on your individual lifestyle and the particular needs of your family and friends.

If you and your partner are expecting a baby, for example, you will find massage and shiatsu a tremendous asset in relieving the aching legs and back and general tiredness that often accompany the later months of pregnancy. And once the child is born, massage will strengthen the bonding between parents and child. It will provide you with a means of soothing and comforting your children that you can return to throughout the growing years – to console them after a bad day at school, to calm them before an exam, or to alleviate minor ailments, such as headaches and tummy pains. Children too should be encouraged to learn massage if they show an interest – by the age of five or six, they have sufficient strength and dexterity in their fingers and often find it most enjoyable.

Many of the occupational hazards of adult life will be greatly alleviated by massage – the aching backs and shoulders incurred after a long stint at the office, the exhaustion or overstrained muscles that result from heavy physical labour or excessive exercise, or the circulatory problems suffered by those who take too little exercise, such as sedentary workers or people who are disabled or bedridden. And for all manner of sports, from cycling to running or football, massage is an invaluable aid, since relaxation is essential for optimum performance.

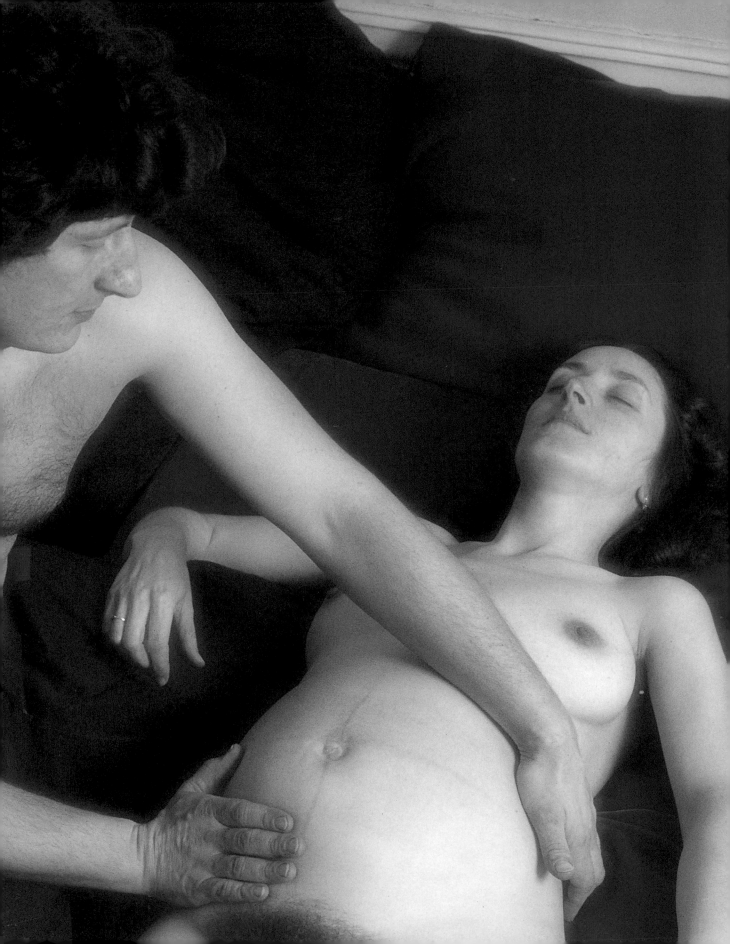

Maternity

Massage is a wonderful way of preparing a woman for childbirth, and helping her to feel more at home with her changing body. It will not only combat tension and fatigue in pregnancy, but will also soothe and reassure a woman in labour. During pregnancy, you can follow the Basic Massage Sequence (pp. 36–7), although in the first four months you should go very gently on the abdomen and avoid pressing deeply around the ankle joints, where points relate to the womb and ovaries. As pregnancy develops and the abdomen starts to swell, it is soothing to rub oil into the area. Use slow, caring strokes, for you are massaging two people at once now. During the labour itself, massage can provide valuable support, as shown below, but try these strokes out before-hand so that you are both accustomed to them well before the birth. And don't forget to use massage after the baby is born – it will help the mother to let go of any stress accumulated during pregnancy and labour. Shiatsu is fine during pregnancy, as long as you avoid deep pressure on the abdomen, and go easy on the leg meridians. During the early stages of labour, it is helpful to press Stomach 36 (p. 128), the "Great Eliminator" (p. 121), and Spleen 6, which is a palm's width above the inner ankle bone, next to the tibia. When the mother begins to bear down, press Gall Bladder 21, which is a tender point halfway along the big muscle on the very top of each shoulder. These points speed delivery and relieve pain. A full reflexology treatment should only be given to expectant mothers by a professional – beginners should concentrate on the relaxation techniques (p. 139).

Alternative Positions

In the later months of pregnancy and in labour, it will no longer be comfort-able for a woman to receive a massage lying flat on her front. For a massage on the back or back of the legs, she should lie on her side with her upper leg propped on a pillow. When she is in this position during labour, you can also help by working on the lower back and buttocks, as shown below left, because contracting muscles in that area may delay the descent of the baby's head. For a front-of-body massage, she may prefer to sit up with her legs apart and her back propped against cushions. With her in this position you can also ease abdominal pressure during labour by lightly stroking the lower belly, beneath the bulge, or relieve trembling legs by stroking the inner thighs, as shown below.

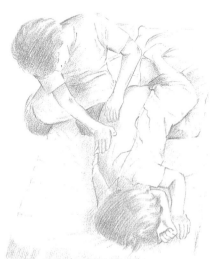

Lower Back and Buttocks

With your partner lying on her side, kneel down by her lower back, facing up the body. Start by circling with your fingers on the lower back and sacrum, then move down to thoroughly knead her buttocks, while she focuses on relaxing these muscles.

Thighs

If your partner's legs start shaking at the end of the first stage of labour, kneel between them and, with your fingers pointing down, mould your hands to the inner thigh and stroke from the upper thigh to the knee and back. Press firmly down the leg and then lightly up, keeping the flow continuous.

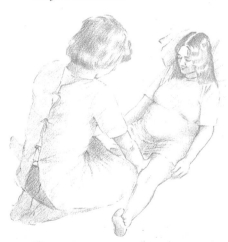

Babies

For both physical and emotional well-being, touch is vital to babies. In many tropical countries, baby massage has always been an integral part of child-rearing – oiling protects the skin from the hot climate, while stroking and stretching the body are commonly believed to help babies grow stronger. (This may well be true, for paediatric research has shown that premature babies progress far more rapidly when regularly massaged.) The sequence we present here is based on the traditional Indian art of massage. It will strengthen the bonding and communication between parent and child and help you to develop your own special way of touching, to calm or comfort your baby. Parents who practise it regularly have found that massage helps babies to sleep and feed better, and relieves colic in the first few months. You can start rubbing your baby lightly with oil from the first week after birth, working up to the full sequence at one month. Try to do the sequence every day, choosing a time when the baby is happy, not tired or hungry – about half an hour after a feed is best. And, ideally, give the baby a warm relaxing bath when you have finished. Don't worry if it takes a little time to get used to the massage – your baby will relax and begin to enjoy it as your touch becomes more confident and assured. As receivers, babies are a challenge, although a rewarding one, for most of them like to take an active part in the proceedings. As your baby wriggles in response to your touch, the massage becomes like a dance, a game between the two of you.

Beginning the Massage

For a baby massage, you need the room to be very warm. It is best to work sitting on the floor, with your legs outstretched. If you need extra support for your back, lean against the wall. You start the massage with your baby lying on your knees, face up and feet pointing toward you. Leave your legs bare so the baby can enjoy more skin contact and lay a towel under you on the floor in case of "accidents". Use a good vegetable oil that is easily absorbed, such as almond or grapeseed, and make sure the oil is warm by standing the bottle in a bowl of hot water. Your hands too should naturally be warm when you come to undress the baby, and any jewellery should be removed. The strokes in the massage sequence work outward from the centre of the body as this is easier and avoids pulling the skin. Try to repeat each stroke at least three times, keeping the rhythm continuous.

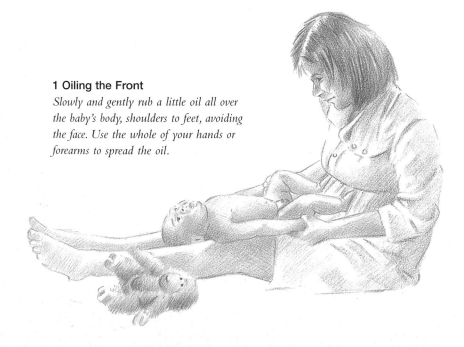

1 Oiling the Front
Slowly and gently rub a little oil all over the baby's body, shoulders to feet, avoiding the face. Use the whole of your hands or forearms to spread the oil.

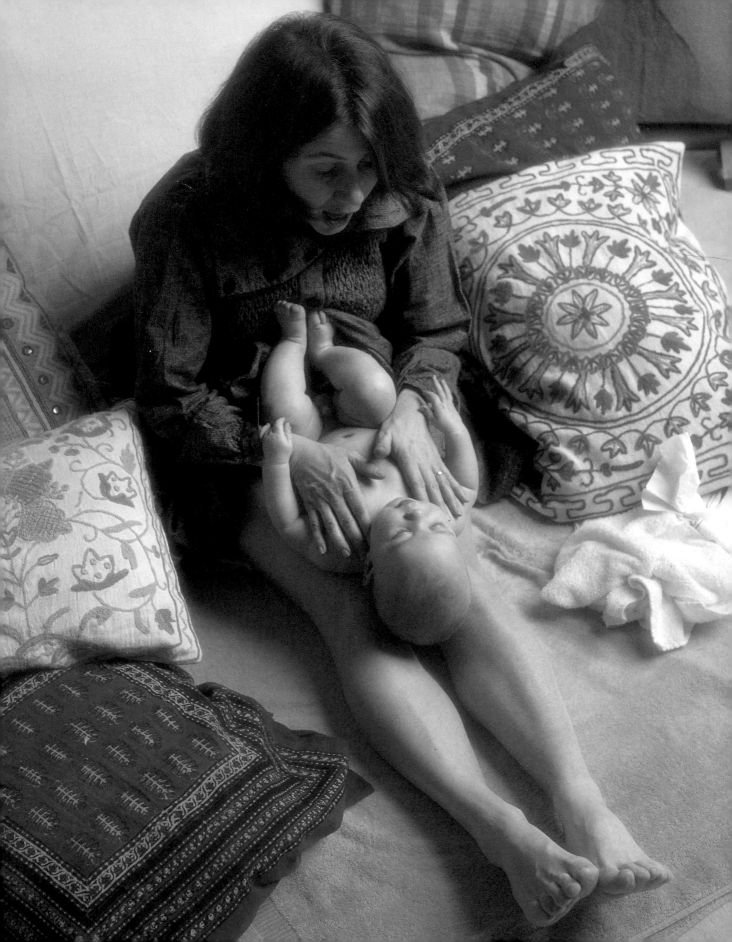

Front of Body

The massage begins on the front of the body, as the baby will feel more relaxed if he or she can see your face, and you can judge from your baby's expressions if you are pressing too firmly or too gently – too light a touch will make the baby feel unsafe. In this sequence you are basically working from the top of the body to the bottom – massaging the chest, arms and hands, then the tummy, legs and feet. Repeat all the strokes three times or so. When massaging the arms and legs, complete one whole limb before starting on the other side.

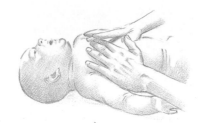

2 "Opening" the Chest

Rest your hands gently on the centre of the chest and begin to circle up and out toward the shoulders, then down the sides of the ribs and back to the centre again.

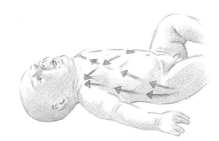

3 Hip and Shoulder Stroking

Start with your hands on either side of the baby's hips. Slide both hands up to meet at the top of the left shoulder, then down again to the sides. Now slide them up to meet on the right shoulder and then back again to the sides.

4 Squeezing and Wringing the Arm

Holding the baby's hand in one of yours, squeeze gently down the arm with your other hand from the wrist to the shoulder, as shown right. Repeat three times. Now clasp the baby's arm in both hands and wring from shoulder to wrist.

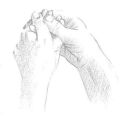

5 "Opening" and Spreading the Hand *(right)*

Use both your thumbs to squeeze the palm open to the sides, as shown right. Now hold the baby's wrist in one hand and slide your free hand slowly across the palm and out over the fingers, unfurling them as you go.

Repeat 4 and 5 on the other arm.

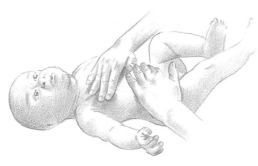

6 Massaging the Tummy *(left)*

Starting on the right side, draw your hands toward you alternately in a continuous stroking movement. Gradually move across the tummy from right to left and back again.

7 Stroking Tummy and Legs

Hold the baby's legs up by the ankles in one hand. Draw your other forearm toward you in a slow sweeping stroke from navel to knees, and back again. Repeat three times, then change hands.

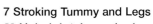

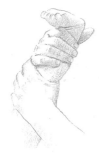

8 Squeezing and Wringing the Leg

Holding the foot in one hand, squeeze the leg from ankle to thigh with the other. Repeat three times, then change hands. Now wring up to the foot, as shown left.

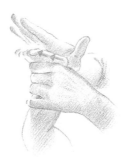

9 "Opening" and Spreading the Foot

Use both your thumbs to squeeze the sole open to the sides. Now hold the baby's ankle or lower leg and slide your palm across the sole from heel to toes, pressing the toes down gently to stretch them.

Repeat 8 and 9 on the other leg.

Back of Body

For this sequence, you lie the baby across your legs on his or her tummy. A back massage is very relaxing for a baby as it soothes the spinal nerves. You begin by massaging up and down the back, and end with some long strokes from top to bottom to "connect" the back and legs. Keep your strokes smooth and flowing, and remember to repeat each one three or four times.

10 Oiling the Back and Legs

Starting at the shoulders, slowly rub a little oil on the back, buttocks, legs and feet. Let your hands enfold the contours of your baby's body as you spread the oil.

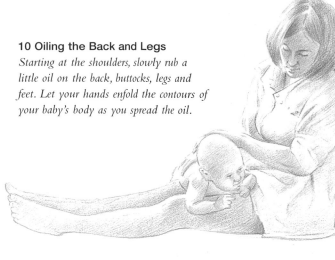

11 Wringing the Back

Start at the baby's bottom with one hand on each side. Now work your way up the back to the shoulders, then down again, crossing your hands repeatedly from one side to the other. Keep your rhythm steady and continuous.

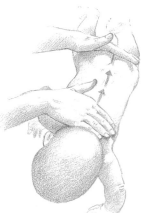

Face

The face sequence is in three parts – first you stroke across the forehead, then across the cheeks, and finish by circling around the mouth. You do each stroke three times or so before moving on to the next. Working around the mouth is good for the sucking muscles. Don't apply any oil to the face and work more lightly here, avoiding the eyes.

12 Stroking the Back

Cup one hand around the baby's bottom and place the other hand on the upper back. Now glide the upper hand firmly down the back to meet the other hand. Squeeze the buttocks gently before lifting your hands off.

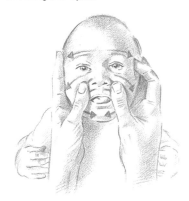

13 Connecting Back and Legs

Hold your baby's ankles in one hand and lift, stretching them a little. Now glide your other hand all the way down the back and legs in a continuous sweep. Lift your hand off. Then place your baby in the original position, to work on the face.

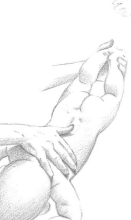

14 Face

A *Place your fingers on the centre of the forehead and slowly draw them out to the side.*

B *Place your fingers on either side of the nose and draw them out to the side, across the cheeks.*

C *Place your thumbs above the upper lip and circle them around the mouth in opposite directions to meet at the chin.*

Later Life

Touch is essential for our well-being at all ages, but at no time do we receive less than in later life. Due to the fear of ageing in our society, the touch that has nurtured and comforted us as children begins to diminish in adulthood and by our later years has dwindled for many to the merest trickle of tenderness or affection. We fail to see that older people are just younger ones in older bodies, that we feel the same person at twelve or seventy, even if we are a little stiffer or slower or have lost the colour of our hair. Massage, shiatsu and reflexology cannot replace a wise and active lifestyle, but used as a supplement to sound nutrition and regular exercise they can greatly enhance the quality of life and combat many of the commonest problems of ageing. All three therapies are calming, relaxing and companionable, helping to relieve high blood pressure, depression and loneliness; all three, given gently, will aid the circulation and alleviate joint pain and muscular stiffness. Massage in particular will keep the skin healthy and pliable, but you should use a good quality oil, such as grapeseed or almond, and moderate your pressure, as the skin tends to get drier and more brittle with age.

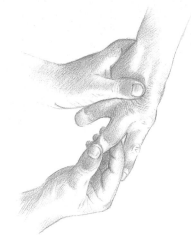

Working on Arthritic Joints
So long as there is no inflammation present, you can ease the stiffness of arthritis by massaging the joints and gently stretching them to their point of resistance, always keeping well within the threshold of pain.

Caution: *Do not massage anyone with cardiovascular problems and only give massage in cases of arthritis when the inflammation has gone.*

Practical Matters

Later in life, it may no longer be comfortable receiving (or giving) a massage on the floor. A massage table is ideal, but if you don't have one, sit your partner in a chair and either give the massage standing up or seated in a chair of a similar height. For a back massage, the receiver can sit astride an upright chair, facing its back and leaning forward against a cushion. Improvise with whatever is available, making sure that you can move freely around your partner. When massaging an older person, have your room warmer than usual and keep a rug handy to cover the parts that you are not actually working on. And let your partner stay dressed, if preferred – a lot can be done by rolling up clothes or even by working through clothing, provided it is not too bulky.

Increasing Flexibility
Many older people suffer from coldness and stiffness in the extremities. Rotating and massaging the wrists and ankles will improve circulation and mobilize the joints. When working on the feet, support the leg so that the knee and foot can relax.

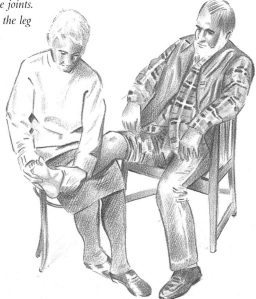

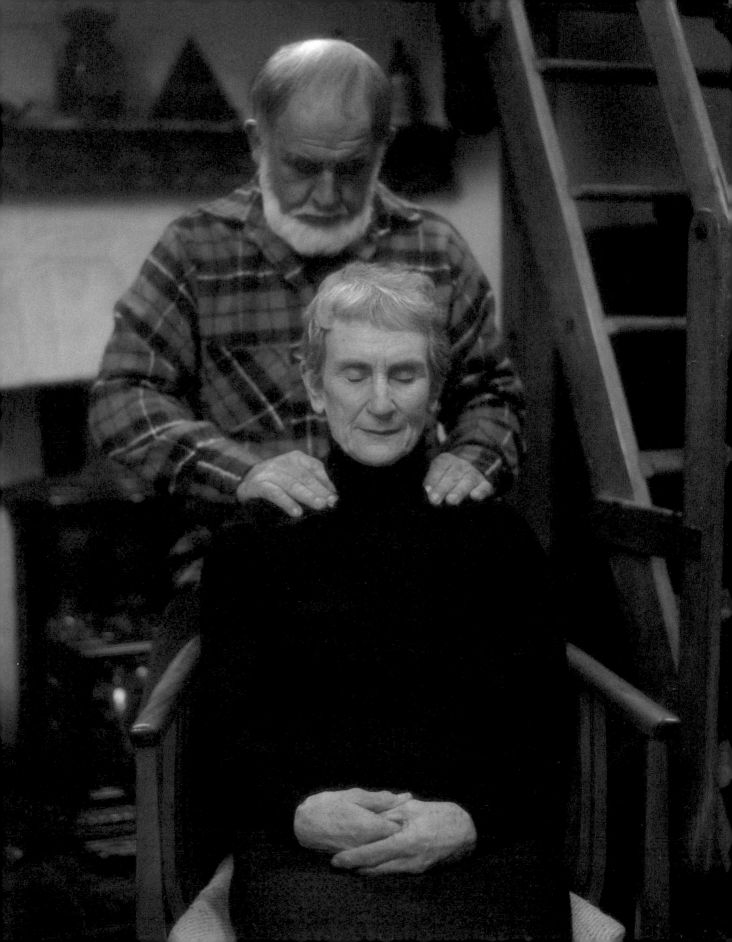

Massage and Exercise

For all forms of exercise, from athletics to dance or cycling, massage is of tremendous value to condition the body for action, relax it, and heal it in times of injury. Before exercise, massage should be used to supplement (but not replace) a warm-up and stretching routine, as shown below. After most forms of exercise, we only need a few moments of rest or panting to restore the metabolic balance in our muscles. But when we are unfit or exercise too hard, the demand for oxygen exceeds the supply, producing a build-up in the muscles of waste products which cause aching and fatigue and take a long time to dispel. Massage helps muscles return to their original capacity far quicker than rest, because it improves circulation and helps remove metabolic wastes. Localized massage will also relieve cramp and fibrositis, and speed the recovery time of muscle or ligament tears, sprains and strains. Reflexology and shiatsu treatments are also most beneficial. Many athletes claim that they run better after a reflexology session, for not only are the feet loosened up but the body is toned and relaxed.

Percussion Strokes

Once you have kneaded the leg muscles quite vigorously, use some percussion strokes such as hacking and pounding to bring extra warmth and stimulation to the area.

Before-exercise Conditioning Massage

A stimulating massage, given preferably the day before any form of strenuous or prolonged exercise, will condition the body and help to prepare it for the coming exertion. If possible your partner should precede the session with a cool shower. You can follow the Basic Massage Sequence (pp. 36–7), but after starting with broad, long strokes, let your pace become brisker than usual and your strokes deeper. Pay special attention to the muscle groups that will be most used, including some kneading and percussion strokes and any of the joint-stretching or mobilization techniques (see pp. 48, 56, 65, and 74). In conditioning the body, you are helping to prevent such problems as cramp and stiffness. After the massage, your partner should rest for half an hour.

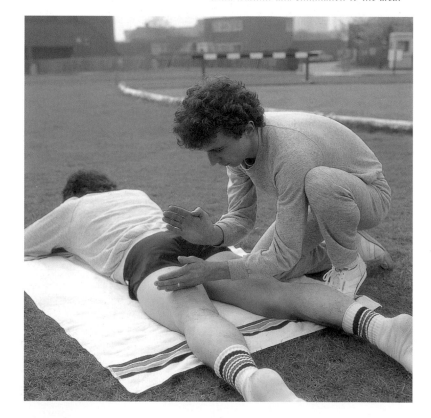

After-exercise Relaxation

The purpose of massage after muscular activity is to help to drain away waste products that may have collected in the tissues and to relax the tired muscles and bring them fresh blood. Ideally, let your partner begin with a warm bath or shower, then cover the body with warmed towels for a few minutes. Have your room very warm, to prevent chilling. As in the massage given before exercise, you should work over the whole body, concentrating on the areas most stressed during exercise, but this time your strokes should be slower and more relaxing.

Begin with long, light strokes and gradually massage more deeply, to drain away metabolic wastes. Work sensitively with any muscles that are sore, or they may try to protect themselves by tightening up even more. If there is any sign of injury, always consult a doctor before massage.

Massage and Exercise Relaxation Strokes

Your aim is to soothe the tired muscles, so use slow, rhythmic draining strokes, working toward the heart to aid the circulation.

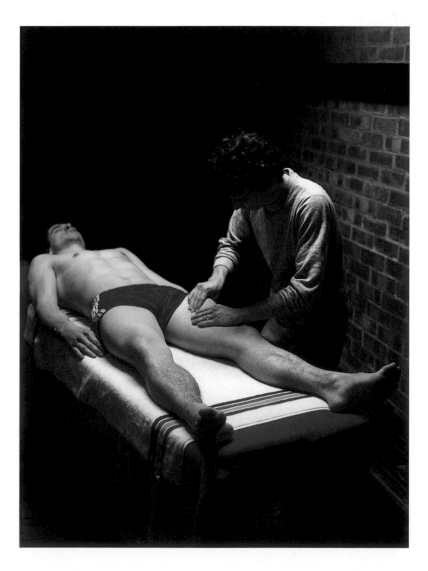

Referral Areas

For anybody who does a lot of sport, dance or other exercise and is liable to muscle damage or strain, it is well worth learning how to treat your own or your friends' injuries using the referral areas of reflexology. Referral areas are parts of the body that correspond to one another anatomically and that can be treated instead of, or as well as, the appropriate injured area. The main ones are the hip and shoulder, the thigh and upper arm, the knee and elbow, the calf and forearm, and the ankle and wrist on the same side of the body. The great value of these referral areas is that when part of the body is hurt or inflamed, you can work on one of them, using the basic thumb technique (see p. 140), instead of on the damaged part. If your partner has a fracture of the right ankle, for example, you can speed up the healing process by treating the corresponding area on the right wrist. Although the referral area itself has not been damaged, it will also feel slightly painful to the touch. The principle works more effectively from the upper to the lower body – in other words it is easier to treat an injured leg by working on the arm than vice versa.

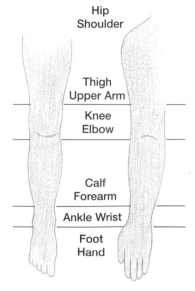

Hip
Shoulder

Thigh
Upper Arm

Knee
Elbow

Calf
Forearm

Ankle Wrist

Foot
Hand

Self-massage

Self-massage is one of the best ways of learning how to be a good masseur, of discovering what feels good in the dual role of giver and receiver. It is an age-old form of healing and one we all turn to instinctively when stiff or in pain – squeezing our tense shoulders or rubbing away a bruise. Many centuries ago, self-massage was used ritualistically by Mongolian warriors, to rid themselves of fear before going into battle. There are drawbacks to self-massage, however, the main ones being the difficulty of relaxing completely and of reaching all parts of the body without straining. But on the whole, any disadvantages are outweighed by the rewards. You can give yourself a massage anywhere - at work, at home or in the car, whenever you feel tense or tired, stiff or aching. Nobody knows your body as well as you do, no-one but you can tell what feels best nor locate so precisely where it hurts.

Self-massage Sequence

You can massage whichever parts of the body you can reach, using any of the strokes in the basic massage sequence. But you will find it easiest to relax if you treat each part in the positions and order shown here, working from feet to head. You can also use these positions to press your own *tsubos* (see p. 131). To give yourself reflexology, sit with one foot over the opposite thigh or, better still, work on your hands (see pp. 148–51). Before you begin, centre yourself in your *hara* (see p. 25). Start each part of the body with a light caress, and gradually work deeper, experimenting with different strokes and pressures. Allow enough time to acquaint yourself fully with each area of your body, so that you emerge feeling restored all over.

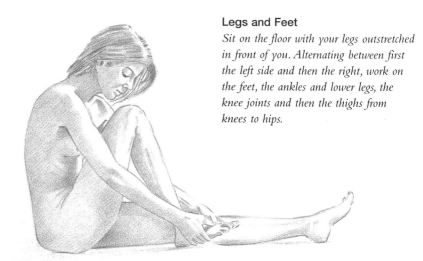

Legs and Feet
Sit on the floor with your legs outstretched in front of you. Alternating between first the left side and then the right, work on the feet, the ankles and lower legs, the knee joints and then the thighs from knees to hips.

Hips and Abdomen
Lie down with your knees up. Massage the whole pelvic area, beginning with the inner triangle from the pubic bone, round between the legs to the sitting bone. Roll over onto one side to work on the area from the sitting bone to the coccyx, over the buttock, and round the pelvic bone and hip joint to the front. Roll over to the other side and repeat. Now massage the entire abdomen.

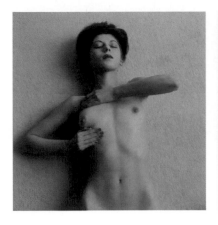 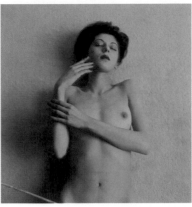 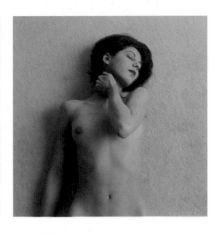

Chest

Lying down, massage from the solar plexus to the collarbone. Pull along the sides of your chest, then work along between the ribs from the midline outward.

Arms and Hands

Lying down, alternate repeatedly between your two arms, starting with the left. First massage each hand, then each forearm including the elbow, and finally the upper arms to the armpits and shoulder joints.

Shoulders and Neck

Lying down, press along the upper edge of the collarbone and the top of the shoulders. Massage the sides and back of the neck and as much of the shoulderblades and upper back as you can reach.

Back

Sitting down, work up from your pelvis as far as you can. Lying down on the floor, wriggle your back against a rolling pin or rubber ball; sitting, roll against a wall; standing, wriggle against a tree.

Face and Scalp

Lying down, stroke the whole face firmly from forehead to chin, working from the centre outward. Massage the jawbone and ears, then the whole scalp.

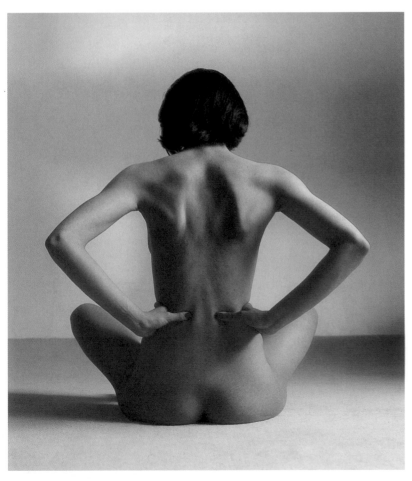

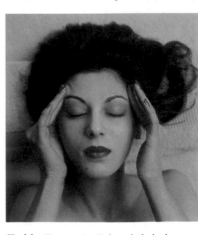

End by "connecting" the whole body, then rest.

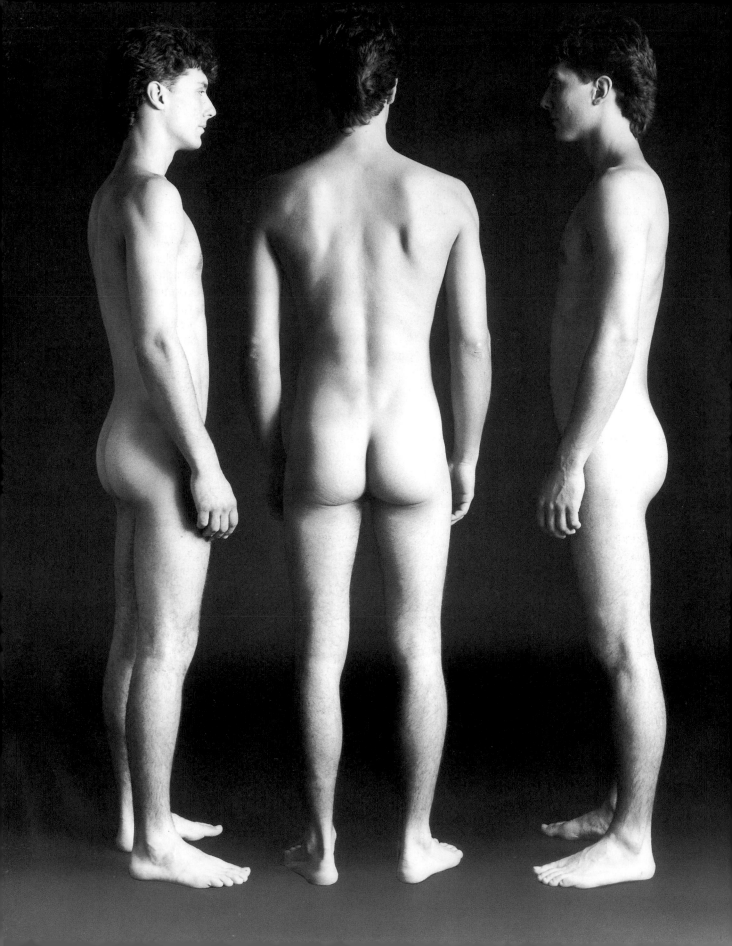

Body Reading

The shape of our bodies is a graphic expression of how we feel and think. It reflects our history, for our structure is moulded by our individual experience of life. Our basic body shape, as well as the separate parts of our frame, reveals a great deal about our psychology – thus a man with the body of a boy may have an unconscious desire to remain a child, while a body that is pale and gaunt may betray an unfulfilled hunger for emotional nourishment. Body reading means understanding the language of the body. It involves interpreting the visual clues that reveal our patterns of feeling, thinking and acting, using this knowledge to help release the tensions that have become embedded in our very fibres.

What are the formative factors that combine to make each one of us unique? We come into the world with aspects of our physical and psycho-logical make-up shaped by the gene pools of our forefathers, but how we then develop as individ-uals is tempered by a variety of other influences: our upbringing; our physical and psychological nourishment in terms of the ideas we take in; how and where we live in the world; our emotional attitudes, occupations and physical activities. Young children need touch and if this need is not supported within the family or if touch is actively discouraged, the child experiences a conflict between wanting to reach out and with-holding the impulse, for fear of rejection. This withholding involves a pattern of muscular contraction which in time becomes chronic and unconscious – manifesting itself perhaps in tight, withdrawn shoulders and arms that hang limply by the sides, unable to reach out for the touch they yearn for, afraid to strive for what they want in life, for fear of failure.

In Oriental medicine, body reading forms a major part of traditional medical diagnosis. Each organ is linked with a specific emotional and mental quality and the doctor picks up clues to the cause of patients' symptoms from the colour of the face, the smell, and voice, as well as from temperature and pulses. In the West, the study and therapeutic uses of the correlation between personality and physical characteristics have been far more recent and it is on these Western systems that our own is based. A wide range of disciplines, including Rolfing and Neo-Reichian therapy, now recognize the important role played by the mind and emotions in the health and structure of the body and involve freeing the personality by working on the body.

The value of body reading is that it provides us with a route map of each individual's problem areas. Having discovered the areas that seem significantly contracted or underdeveloped, say, or those where the energy seems stagnant or excessive, you can try to balance and harmonize the structure. In general you will be concentrating on releasing tight areas from tension – in the case of reflexology, by paying special attention to the painful reflexes; in massage, by gradually working more deeply into blocked or held areas.

In this chapter we are only able to present some extreme ways in which our approach to life is shown in various parts of the body, but most people will exhibit far subtler variations from "normal". When looking at your own or another's body, don't fall into the trap of making glib gener-alizations from isolated structural patterns. Body reading is a skill that is developed with practice and calls for a compassionate, non-judgemental attitude. The more bodies you look at in this way, the more you learn to use your intuition to obtain an accurate picture. Each person is unique – and the whole may give a very different message than the sum of its parts.

Splits and Asymmetries

When you read a body for the first time, you should begin by trying to get an overall impression rather than concentrating on specific areas. Start by spending a few moments centring yourself, with your eyes closed (see p. 25). Then open your eyes and allow yourself to be receptive to whatever captures your attention. You might be struck by differences in colour or texture – one area of the body may look healthy and glowing, another paler and less alive. See what shape and size the body is. Is it basically tall and thin, say, or short and muscular? Where is the energy focused? Is the general impression powerful and strong or weak and tentative? You may notice that the lines of the body flow smoothly or that the figure seems disjointed, disproportionately large in some places and small in others. One part of the body may not seem to fit with the rest – perhaps the head appears large, or the top and bottom halves look as though they belong to two different people. You will often find that the body looks split into two different areas. The most frequently encountered splits and asymmetries are top/bottom, left/right, and front/back.

Top-heavy (below left)
The overinflated upper half looks as if it is compensating for a feeling of insecurity at the base. The hips and legs look underdeveloped by comparison with the top part.

Well-balanced (below centre)
Weight is evenly distributed between the top and bottom halves. Energy appears to flow smoothly up and down the body, with no sense of constriction in the middle.

Bottom-heavy (below right)
The legs and hips are oversized by comparison with the upper half. Her stance seems almost defiant, but the chest area appears withdrawn and constricted.

Top/Bottom Split

In a top/bottom split, the energy and vitality of the body seem to be displaced upward or downward, so that the body looks top-or bottom-heavy. It is as if the energy is blocked at some level, causing an over-abundance of energy at one end and a mere trickle at the other. The part that lacks vitality will be noticeably paler and weaker and often feel cooler to the touch. In a person who is top-heavy, the chest and shoulders look inflated but the pelvis and legs appear tight and underdeveloped. In someone who is bottom-heavy, the legs are large and heavy, but the upper half is contracted and narrow. Top-heavy people are likely to be assertive, rationally orientated, and active; they are most often male. Bottom-heavy people tend to be passive and find it hard to assert themselves. More at home on a feeling level, they are most often female.

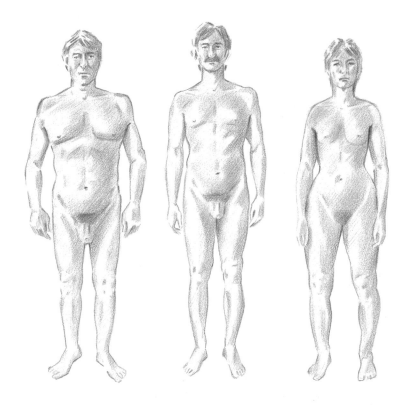

Left/Right Split

Nobody is totally symmetrical, but some people display a striking degree of asymmetry. This can be due to structural imbalances such as scoliosis or tilting of the hips. There may also be a difference in the musculature of the two sides – one may be harder and more angular, say, the other softer and rounder. The left side of the body is mainly controlled by the right hemisphere of the cerebral cortex, and vice versa. Recent scientific research has found that the left brain is primarily concerned with rational, linear thought and verbal functioning, and the right with the more intuitive, visuo-spatial, emotional side of life. The two sides of the body may reflect this distinction. But if the person is well balanced, the body will evolve symmetrically. Pronounced asymmetry suggests conflict – perhaps between reason and emotion.

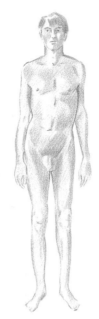 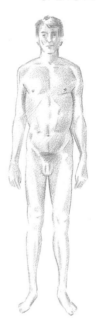 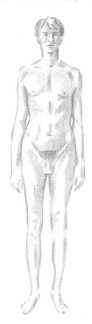

Left/Right Split
This man shows a fairly pronounced split, with the hips and shoulders tilted, so that the left is higher. The discrepancy is clearer in the composite pictures of the two sides, right.

Left Composite
The figure seems quite strong and tall, with the energy displaced upward. He stands upright and appears resolute and ready for action.

Right Composite
The figure is softer and more rounded at the hips, making it more feminine. The shoulders are lower and the energy displaced downward. He seems more passive.

Front/Back Split

A front/back split occurs when someone seems to present a different character when seen from behind than he or she does from the front. The front of the body represents the way we wish to be seen, the "front" we consciously project to the world. The back reflects our more unconscious side, aspects of our personality that we may be hiding from the world or from ourselves. Normally you will find that the back manifests more tension and negativity, like a cellar in which we store things we have forgotten.

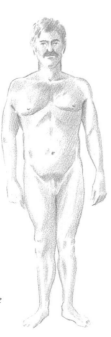 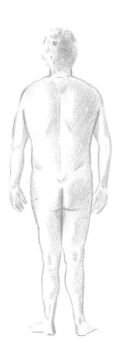

Back of Body
From the back he seems crushed and rather sad. Although his shoulders are broad, they seem overburdened and his legs look weaker.

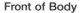

Front of Body
From the front, this man appears quite strong and powerful. His stance and shoulder position are defiant.

Feet and Legs

The state of our feet and legs reflects our relationship with reality, the condition of our Root Chakra (see p. 189) and our foundations – our earliest experiences of various kinds of "support", from the womb to our mother's arms and the ground or "mother earth" itself. As two-legged animals we make contact with the earth's energy field through our feet. We either "stand our ground" or are "push-overs"; we can be "weak-kneed" or learn to "stand on our own two feet". Expressions like these reflect our instinctive understanding of the link between the feet and the legs and our whole sense of security, confidence and contact with reality – the earth on which we walk. Insecurity may be expressed through weak legs and feet, the muscles undeveloped and flaccid, unequal to the task of bearing our weight. Or we may compensate for insecurity by stiffening our legs and feet, making the muscles hard and the joints tightly locked.

Grounding

In order for energy to flow unimpeded through the body, good contact with the ground is essential. Ungrounded people tend to be unsure of their footing or hold on reality. Their muscles may be either rigid or flaccid – both inadequate when faced with new terrain. These physical characteristics may accompany corresponding mental attitudes of rigidity or laxity. Grounded people seem well balanced and aligned. With their flexible feet and legs they adjust quickly to unfamiliar terrain, and remain open and responsive to any new input in their lives.

Feet

It is with our feet that we make contact with the ground, exchanging energy with the earth like the roots of a tree. To understand the part your feet play, stand up and spend a few minutes sensing them with your shoes off. Check how your weight is distributed – toward the balls, the heels or the sides? Do you feel comfortable on your feet? Are you tense or relaxed? Perhaps your weight is mainly on the insides, with your arches dropped, in an attempt to get more purchase on the floor. Or maybe your feet look fairly relaxed with well-curved arches at the instep supporting your weight without strain. Alternatively, you might notice that your feet seem cramped, with a high, rigid instep and toes curled round. Illustrated right are the three types of feet you will encounter most frequently.

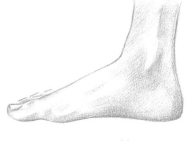

Flat Foot

The arches are collapsed, weakening the structure. The foot appears to be trying to cling to the ground for extra support. The weight is generally thrown toward the inside of the ankles.

"Normal" Foot

Here, the whole foot has a supple quality – the weight is evenly distributed on balls and heels and the supportive arch can be seen at the centre of the inner foot.

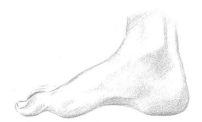

Rigid Foot

The foot appears tight and excessively contracted, making precarious contact with the ground. The arches under the toes and instep are pulled tightly upward; the toes may be curled under, as if trying to claw into the earth.

Ankles and Knees

Like the feet, the ankles and knees are connected with grounding, mobility and balance. Any imbalance or weakness in the feet may affect these joints too. The way people walk reveals a lot about their self-image and hold on reality – from swaggering to scurrying or striding. If the ankles are misaligned or weak, the steps may be tentative and faltering. The knees relate especially to our sense of security – when we are scared, our knees will tremble. In the long term, insecurity will reflect in the knees being braced in defiance or determination or in an effort to stop oneself falling or failing.

Normal and Locked Knees

The "normal" knee (right) is supple and relaxed, allowing energy to flow directly up and down the centre of the leg. The pulled back knee (far right) looks rigid, blocking the energy flow and making movement stiff.

Thigh and Leg Shapes

Our capacity for sustained effort and activity and our sexuality are reflected in the thighs. When we feel threatened, the legs are charged with energy as we prepare for fight or flight. If no action is taken, the legs may shake with fear as the energy attempts to discharge itself. In some people, chronic insecurity and inability to take action manifest themselves in a characteristic shape of the legs – they may be heavy and flaccid, for instance, or tight and rigid, or weak and undeveloped as if resigned to their situation. Two common stances are shown right.

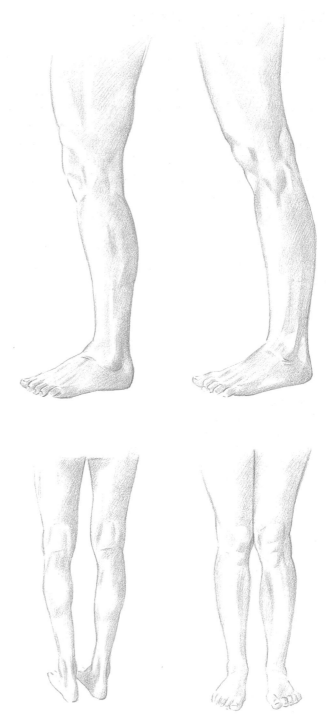

Bow Legs and Knock Knees

Bow legs (above left) culminate in a high peak with the thigh muscles pulled in and up toward the genitals, impeding pelvic mobility and hence full sexual expression. A knock-kneed stance *(above right) reflects a self-protective attitude, as the legs press together for support. Here too sexual vitality may be limited, as the genitals are squeezed by the thighs.*

The Pelvis

The pelvis is a bowl-shaped structure that joins the legs to the torso and supports the spine. Its major joints at the hips and the base of the spine facilitate mobility in the whole body, especially walking. The entire pelvic area is linked to the Root Chakra and *hara*, and nerves from the lower spine activate the sexual and eliminative functions, as well as the legs and feet. As we have seen, tension and imbalance in one area of the body reflect back onto other areas by way of muscular compensation, thus pelvic stiffness may result from ungrounded legs and vice versa. The way we use and move our hips expresses our attitudes to sex and elimination. A pelvis that is not "blocked" can swing freely back and forth when we move, but a pelvis that is full of tension moves as one solid block, causing the legs also to move stiffly. Tension in this area may affect the buttocks too and often indicates lack of full sexual expression.

The Tilted Pelvis

Tilted forward (below left), the buttocks are pulled in and the pelvis thrust forward and up. This position is often accompanied by weak or rigid legs and an overdeveloped upper half of the body. Tilted back (below right), the lower back is tight and hollow, the buttocks are thrust out, and the pelvis is pulled back like a drawn bow. It is as if the person is frightened of letting go.

The Tilted Pelvis

When a lot of tension and energy are held in the pelvic area, not only will the range of movement be limited, but the pelvis is often held habitually in a forward or backward tilt. In the "thrust forward" position (right), the pelvis appears unable to swing back to gather fresh energy for a renewed thrust and open release of feelings. In the retracted position (far right), the pelvis is highly charged but may be unable to swing forward to release the charge, resulting in pent-up energy.

Buttocks

The buttock muscles attach the pelvis to the legs and help to define their relative positions and range of movement. Tension in this part may reflect problems with giving and receiving and a need for possession. The area is connected with elimination. If children are toilet trained too early, other muscles such as those of the pelvic floor and buttocks can be brought into play to control bowel movements. This tightening may be carried forward unconsciously into adult life.

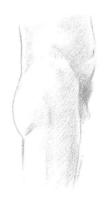
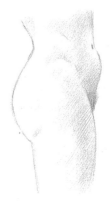
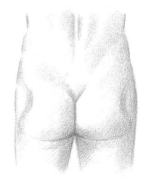
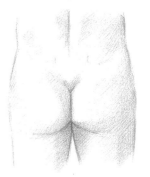
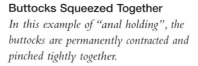

Buttocks Squeezed Together
In this example of "anal holding", the buttocks are permanently contracted and pinched tightly together.

Pelvic Floor Pulled Up
Here the inner thigh muscles are pulled up and the muscles of the pelvic floor – the pubococcygeal muscles – are tightened.

The Belly

The belly is the seat of the *hara*, our centre of gravity, strength and vitality and is closely linked with our legs and our sense of grounding. It houses our gut feelings, the instinctual drives of hunger, sexuality and emotional fullness or emptiness and, if we breathe freely and deeply, it moves with our breath. Western culture, however, does not look kindly on the belly unless it is flat and firm, and constricts it with belts and corsets if its own muscles are not strong enough to hold it in. In the process, our gut feelings are stifled and, cut off from our most primitive drives, our heads assume control, often disregarding our basic needs. Between the head and the belly lies the heart, our emotional centre, which becomes entangled in the conflicting pulls of gut feelings and reason. Only when all three centres work in harmony can we achieve integration and balance.

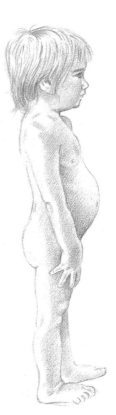

The Estranged Belly

One way in which many people cut themselves off from their bellies is by pulling the abdominal muscles in and keeping them contracted. This reaction is often found in those who adopt the military "chin up, chest out, belly in" stance. Lack of contact with the belly's needs may also be demonstrated by obesity, where we try mistakenly to compensate for feeling empty by overeating when in fact the sense of emptiness is often engendered by being separated from our gut feelings.

Natural Belly *(right)*
In young children and people of "primitive" societies, the abdominal wall is generally relaxed and the belly expands freely with every inhalation. Belly and chest are integrated, rather than separate.

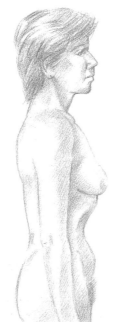

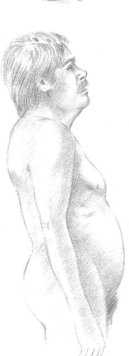

Taut Belly *(right)*
Here the belly is constantly pulled in, the muscles are hard and rigid, and the basic drives restrained. This type of armouring also restricts an individual to shallow chest breathing.

Bloated Belly *(far right)*
An obese, heavy belly may cover and hide the feelings within. Out of touch with this vital centre, this individual may be unable to recognize and fulfil his needs.

The Chest

In its natural state, the chest is a flexible bony cage, constantly undulating with the rhythm of our breath. It contains and protects the vital organs of heart and lungs, and is related to the Solar Plexus, Heart and Throat Chakras – the centres of vital energy or consciousness concerned with energy intake and distribution, emotion, and the expression of feelings (see p. 189). In a person whose chest area moves easily, without armouring, the tenderness and warmth associated with the heart can be exchanged freely; but where energy here is blocked, as a protection against hurt, such feelings are less easily expressed. The diaphragm is the main respiratory muscle. It spreads horizontally from the front to the back of the ribcage and, if it is flexible, massages the abdominal organs, the heart and the lungs as it rises and falls. Full, relaxed breathing energizes and nourishes the whole body, but all too often the energy flow is blocked. If our feelings are too painful we learn to tighten the breathing muscles unconsciously, since restricting one's breath is a way of deadening feelings.

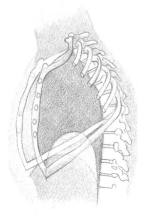

Normal Respiration

When we inhale, the diaphragm contracts and moves down, pulling the lower ribs and breastbone up and out, aided by the intercostal muscles, and the abdomen begins to swell. As the ribs rise, they enlarge the chest cavity, which causes air to be drawn into the lungs. As the diaphragm relaxes and moves, the elastic wall of the chest recoils and air is expelled from the lungs.

Overexpanded and Collapsed Chests

Our chests are capable of containing great intensity of feeling, but when the diaphragm is habitually tightened, limiting our breathing, we starve ourselves of vitality, both physical and emotional. Chronic tension can result in a variety of response patterns, of which the two extremes are the over-expanded and the collapsed chest. Individuals with overexpanded chests appear to have an inflated upper body, often dwindling down to an under-developed lower half. As personalities they can seem rational, assertive and self-sufficient. But in reality they are defensive and scared of letting go. By contrast, those with collapsed or deflated chests are unable to inhale deeply, to recharge their energy. As a result, they look pale and weary and frequently seem withdrawn and in need of support.

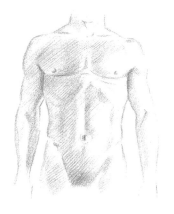

Overexpanded Chest

The chest looks puffed up and raised. Its rigid muscles prevent it from moving much on an exhalation. Loosening the chest muscles can help counteract this pattern and allow a full exhalation.

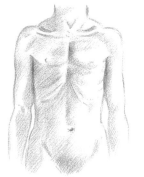

Collapsed Chest

The chest looks taut and fragile, as if it has caved in. People with this kind of chest seem resigned and hurt. If they can learn to breathe deeply, they can re-experience and integrate their pain and regain their energy.

Shoulders and Arms

Our shoulders and arms are associated with work, action, responsibility, and how we relate to the outside world. With our upright posture freeing the upper limbs from the ground, and the development of a thumb that we can place in opposition to all the other fingers, we are uniquely equipped among living creatures for a wide spectrum of activities – for wielding tools and weapons, giving and getting, striking or embracing. Through the shoulders and arms, many emotions are expressed or inhibited – emotions that arise in the belly and the chest, with which the shoulders are closely related. The energy centre linked to this area is the Throat Chakra, which is primarily concerned with self-expression and communication, via the arms or voice. Try acting out a range of feelings, such as anger, joy, superiority, fear, despair and so forth and notice the part played by your shoulders in expressing these emotional attitudes.

Shoulders and Arms

The way we hold our shoulders and the degree of mobility in our arms often reveal unresolved emotions. Among the most common positions are pulled forward or hunched shoulders, that usually signify a self-protective attitude, pulled back shoulders, associated with suppressed anger, and shoulders that are raised in an habitual expression of fear. Heredity may also predispose us to a shoulder shape that reflects a certain way of relating, of shouldering or relinquishing responsibilities. Of these, two types are shown – overdeveloped and narrow.

Raised Shoulders

Frozen by fear (right), the shoulders remain raised while head and neck cower down in them for safety.

Shoulders Pulled Back

The shoulders are retracted (centre right), as if to restrain the individual from striking out. The neck and lower jaw are thrust defiantly forward and the arms pulled out to the sides.

Shoulders Pulled Forward

The shoulders curve around protectively (far right), as if to guard the chest and heart. In this position, the ribcage is often contracted and the upper chest withdrawn, with the arms squeezed in to the sides.

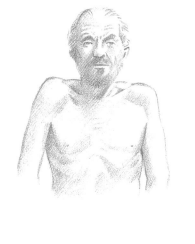 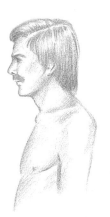 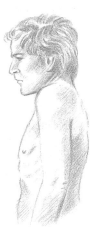

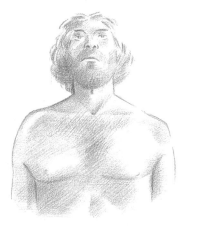 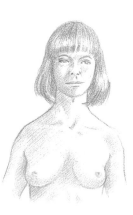

Overdeveloped Shoulders

Strong broad shoulders are generally associated with the male stereotype. When they are also rounded they indicate a personality that feels overburdened (far left). The arms are often rotated inward, like a gorilla's.

Narrow Shoulders

Besides being slight, the shoulders often droop and look compressed (left), indicating that the individual cannot shoulder her responsibilities and lacks the energy to cope or effect change. The arms may also hang limply.

Neck, Head, and Face

In the region of the neck and head, the Throat, Brow and Crown Chakras are located – the energy centres that relate to self-expression and communication, self-awareness, and superconsciousness (see p. 189). The neck is a busy thoroughfare for the transport of blood to the brain and air to the lungs and a passageway that mediates between our thoughts and our feelings in the form of nerve impulses. Along with the throat, it is a common site of tension and constriction if we feel emotionally overloaded. In terms of body reading, the face is among the most revealing parts of the body and possibly the easiest to "read". Expression is a statement of experience and often our faces shape themselves around one central theme – a theme that is either a true reflection of our feelings or a mask we have chosen as a disguise to confront the world outside. Many of us choose a mask of innocence, say, or superiority, in order to create a specific impression and, more importantly, to obtain a certain response – perhaps to give ourselves satisfaction for the unfulfilled needs of childhood we still carry with us.

Head and Neck

The way you carry your head is expressive of how you feel about yourself and the world at large. If you are open and relaxed, the neck will be supple and mobile and the head sit centrally over the body. But more often the neck is chronically tense and, over a period of time, the neck and head become fixed in a characteristic position. A head that pokes forward may indicate an aggressive or determined quality, but in conjunction with an over-curved spine it suggest collapse and, often, longing, loneliness or depression. When the head and neck are pulled back (right), it can signify an inflexible personality and someone who is more of a doing than feeling person.

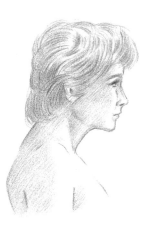

Head Thrust Forward
The head pokes out ahead of the rest of the body (below left), giving either an aggressive impression or one of neediness and dependence, as here. The attitude is often reinforced by the jaw jutting forward too.

Head Pulled Back
When head and neck are retracted (bottom left), the posture may indicate a rigid, achievement-orientated outlook.

Head Tilted to the Side
A head that leans to one side (below), suggests indecision, an inability to confront life directly or "head-on". If the head is also bowed, it indicates a certain coyness.

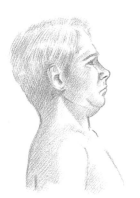

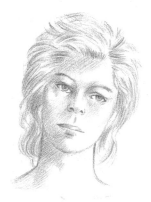

The Face

Like the rest of the body, much of the structure of the face and its expressions are shaped by emotional and mental attitudes. For the purpose of interpreting the face, you can usefully divide it into three main sections. The area above the eyebrows is the mental and spiritual section; the area on either side of the nose, including the eyes, is the emotional section; and the oral area, from the nostrils downward, relates more to the physical and sexual aspects of the body, especially to energy intake. The general shape and character of the different features also mirror the parts of the body, as shown on the face map, right. As you can see, the jaw corresponds to the pelvis, and tension in one is often echoed in the other. A clenched jaw may be suppressing anger, and is scared of losing control and letting go; a tight pelvis is often holding back from being sexually assertive. A protruding, overdeveloped jaw denotes determination and defiance, while a receding, underdeveloped jaw may indicate a withdrawn approach to life, as shown right. The mouth itself expresses how needy or fulfilled we are in terms of emotional and physical nourishment – the lips may be full and relaxed, say, or thin and tight. The eyes are said to be the windows of the soul and, in fact, the retina of the eye is derived from brain tissue. No other features boast such a versatility of expressions – from withering or piercing to loving, trusting or beseeching. In many faces, you will observe a left/right split between the two eyes. In esoteric philosophy, the right and left eyes are said to possess different energies. The right eye signifies the ego, activity, maleness, and relationship with the father; the left eye signifies essence or spirit, receptivity, femaleness and relationship with the mother.

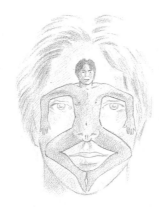

Face Map

The various features of the face relate to different parts of the body, acting like a map. The forehead corresponds with the head and the eyebrows with the shoulders and arms. The centre of the face represents the torso, the eyes being on a level with the heart. The tip of the nose corresponds to the hara, *the mouth to the genitals, the jaw and chin to the pelvis, legs and feet.*

Protruding, Overdeveloped Jaw

The jaw is thrust forward in an expression of aggression and obstinacy.

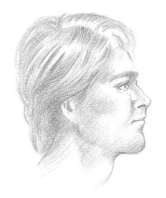

Receding, Underdeveloped Jaw

The jaw wears a hurt expression, as if the individual has been constantly rebuffed and feels unable to "speak out".

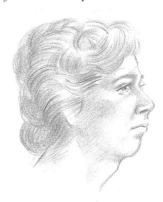

Left and Right Eye Imbalance

The right eye appears more open and outgoing, while the left eye looks more tense, closed and defensive.

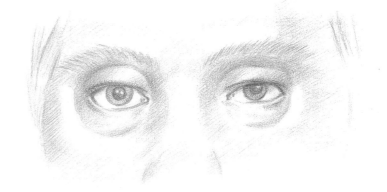

The Body Speaks

Our bodies tell the story of our lives – our fears and aspirations, our deepest secrets and experiences. Each one is unique, a world of its own making, comparable only to itself. Here we look at three different bodies to show you how you might set about distilling your impressions, bringing the various signals together and viewing the person as a whole. If you want to start by reading your own body, you can either stand in front of a large mirror, using a small hand-held mirror to show you your back or, better still, arrange two large mirrors at an angle so that you can see two sides at once. When you come to read the bodies of your friends, observe their movements and postures before they lie down, how they use their bodies, the way they breathe. Once they are lying flat, you can round off your first impressions by seeing how well the body melts down on to the working surface or whether parts are held up by tension. Be careful not to project your own preconceptions of how you think it should look. Listen to the body, let it speak to you, without making judgements or comparisons. Share what you find with your partner and use your discoveries to guide your hands, to help release the body from its armour.

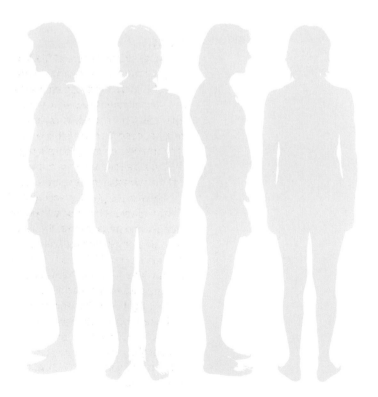

Joe

Joe's body looks compressed, as if he has been squashed down. In fact, when he looks at himself in a mirror, he is surprised to see that he is larger than he thought, for he feels smaller than he actually is. His body gives the impression of being resigned and constrained, especially in the chest area. There is a feeling of congestion around the pelvis and belly area and from the side it is evident that the pelvis is strongly retracted and the lower back hollow. The shoulders too are pulled back and also slightly raised, suggesting a mixture of fear and lack of self-assertion. Joe's upper chest is contracted and needs to open out. Deep breathing would help to loosen the habitual tension and congestion of the chest and abdomen.

Sue

In both the front and back views, Sue's stance is that of a little girl, defenceless and slightly questioning. The feet are flat and overgrounded, and the legs, though quite well developed, look a little forlorn. The pelvis is retracted and twisted backward to the right. Most of her energy seems to have gathered in the belly, hips and legs which look fuller and stronger than the upper half. The chest, by comparison, is tight and contracted and her shoulders, neck and jaw seem tense. From the side you can see that her head is forward – in fact the whole upper half of the body seems ready to go forward, while the lower half holds back and hesitates. This impression of uncertainty is emphasized by the legs and arms – the left arm and foot are ahead, the right behind.

Mark

The most striking feature of Mark's body is the left/right split. The whole right side looks more compressed and taut – the ribcage leans down to the right, the right shoulder is lower and more rounded than the left and the right arm consequently looks longer. The hips are tilted up toward the right and the weight is mainly on the right leg. There is a slight displacement of energy upward – the top half seems stronger and more mature, the legs look more boyish and undeveloped. The head is held high, like a soldier on parade. The overriding impression of the whole figure is a readiness for "fight or flight" – particularly from the front, Mark looks both challenging and a little defensive. His general rigidity and uptight stance may mask a fear of letting go, of getting in touch with his softer, gentler side.

Anatomy

When you are new to massage it is better to learn about the structure of the body by touch before acquiring an intellectual understanding of anatomy. If you practise the basic sequence of strokes on your own and others' bodies, you will soon begin to get a sense of the framework underlying the skin beneath your hands. Once your interest is stimulated to look into the structure and workings of the body, you will find it adds a rich new dimension to the knowledge you have gained by experience. In this chapter we present you with a glimpse of the body's anatomy and physiology, travelling from the architecture of bones and muscles to the nervous system and skin, and finally to the aura or "subtle energy" bodies that surround our physical body.

Skeleton

Over 200 bones make up the skeleton (see opposite), the flexible framework of the body. The bones not only support the body and protect some of the most delicate organs, they also make movement possible, acting as levers at the joints or the points of connection between them. The ridges which can be seen on some of the bone surfaces opposite are for the attachment of muscles.

Anatomy of a Bone

All bones are moist and active, and require nourishment, like any living organ. They consist of a hard outer covering and a porous inner portion – the bone marrow – which contains the rich blood supply that brings them all the nutrients they need. Bone marrow manufactures red blood cells and serves as an important mineral reserve. The structure of a long bone, such as the thigh or femur, is shown right.

Hard Bone

Spongy Medulla

Nutrient Artery

Marrow Cavity

Joints

When two or more bones of the skeleton meet, a joint is formed. In structure and function, joints vary enormously from freely moving ones like those in the limbs, to ones that are immobile like those that link the bones of the skull. There are several kinds of free-moving joint, including the hinge joints, such as the knees, ankles, and elbows, and the ball-and-socket types such as the hip and shoulder joints. The ends of the bones in free-moving joints are covered with cartilage and linked by a fibrous capsule, lined with a smooth tissue called synovial membrane which secretes the joints' lubricant – synovial fluid. Production of this fluid is stimulated by massage.

The Knee
The knee is the body's largest joint. It is a hinge joint that can move in one plane only, like the hinge of a door.

The Hip
Like all ball-and-socket joints, the hip has a round head that fits into a cupped socket, allowing movement in any direction.

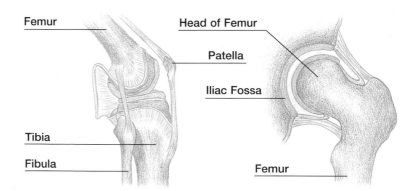

Femur

Head of Femur

Patella

Iliac Fossa

Tibia

Fibula

Femur

Front View

Back View

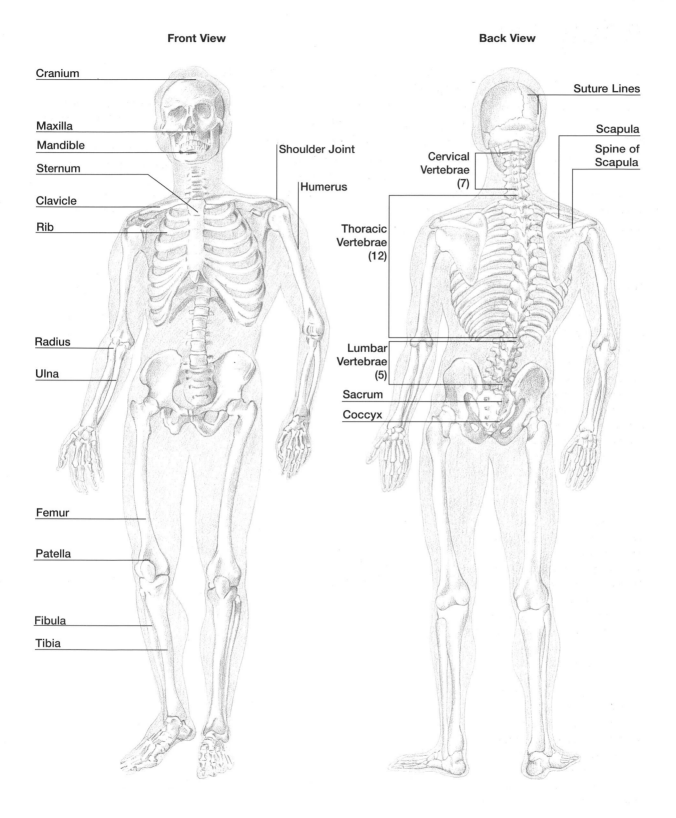

Cranium

Maxilla

Mandible

Sternum

Clavicle

Rib

Radius

Ulna

Femur

Patella

Fibula

Tibia

Shoulder Joint

Humerus

Suture Lines

Scapula

Spine of Scapula

Cervical Vertebrae (7)

Thoracic Vertebrae (12)

Lumbar Vertebrae (5)

Sacrum

Coccyx

Muscles

Muscles enable us to move, and contribute to our shape, as well as helping us to breathe, digest food, circulate blood, and perform innumerable other body functions. There are two main types: the skeletal muscles that you can move voluntarily, and the involuntary muscles, like those of the heart, which move automatically. Each end of a skeletal muscle is attached to a bone on either side of a joint. Most muscles move in pairs, one moving the joint in one direction, the other moving it in the opposite direction. The skeletal muscles are ranged in layers, and placed symmetrically on each side of the body. In the illustrations opposite, the superficial layer of muscles has been removed from the right-hand side of the body, to expose the deepest layer beneath. Massage can help to dispel the hard knots of muscular spasm, caused by chronic tension or emotional or physical trauma.

Structure of Muscles

Muscles are made up of overlapping bundles of fibres or cells, supplied with blood, lymph and nerves. Tendons at the ends of a muscle attach it to bones. The fullest part of a muscle is the centre, known as the "belly". Its two ends are called the origin, at the anchoring point, and the "insertion", at the pulling point. The bundles of fibres in the belly of a muscle are made up of even smaller bundles of fibrils or filaments that are capable of contraction (see right).

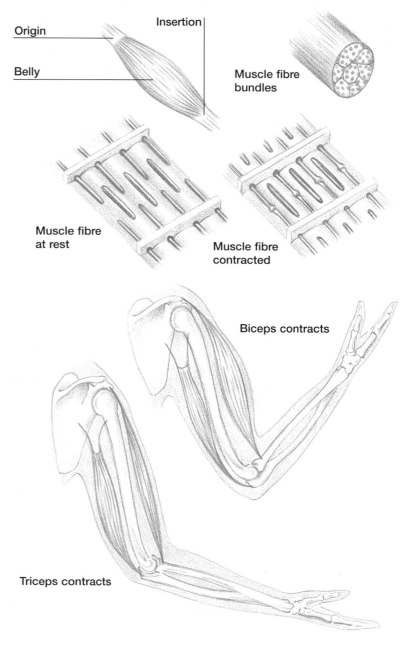

Origin

Belly

Insertion

Muscle fibre bundles

Muscle fibre at rest

Muscle fibre contracted

Biceps contracts

Triceps contracts

Function of Muscles

When a muscle receives a message from the brain to contract, the fibres slide between one another, as shown above right, causing the whole muscle to swell and shorten. This in turn causes the bones to which the muscle is attached to be drawn closer together, effecting movement. Muscles that bend joints are called flexors, while those that straighten them are called extensors. When you bend your elbow, for example, the biceps – the flexor muscle on the front of the upper arm – contracts and raises the radius, the bone of the forearm. When you lower your arm the triceps – the extensor muscle on the back of the upper arm – contracts and the biceps relaxes and stretches, as shown right.

Front View

Back View

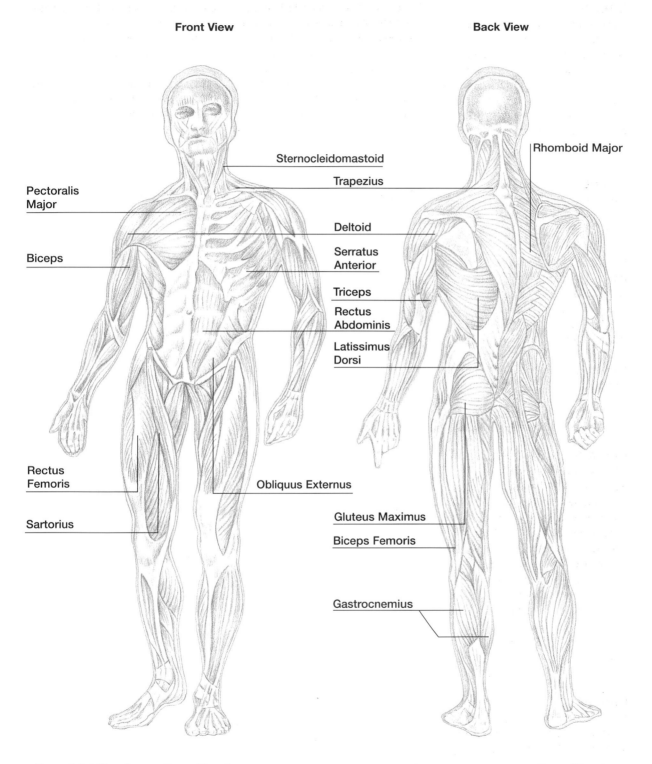

Sternocleidomastoid

Trapezius

Rhomboid Major

Pectoralis
Major

Deltoid

Biceps

Serratus
Anterior

Triceps

Rectus
Abdominis

Latissimus
Dorsi

Rectus
Femoris

Obliquus Externus

Sartorius

Gluteus Maximus

Biceps Femoris

Gastrocnemius

Superficial Muscles **Deep Muscles**

Superficial Muscles **Deep Muscles**

Circulation

The circulatory system transports the blood round and round the body – hence its name, circulation. As the blood circulates, it carries oxygen and other nutrients to the cells, removes waste products, and destroys invading bacteria with its white corpuscles. The system is driven by the heart, a highly efficient muscular pump which transports about 6 litres (10½ pints) of blood per minute when the body is at rest, up to 24 litres (42 pints) during strenuous exercise. The adult body contains about 7 litres (12 pints) of blood, so even when resting all our blood makes a complete circulation in just over a minute. The bright red oxygenated blood is pumped out by the heart and travels through the arteries of the body, ending in tiny blood vessels called capillaries, where the oxygen and nutrients are exchanged for carbon dioxide and other waste products. Now darker in colour, the waste-laden blood returns via the veins to the heart where it is pumped through to the lungs for purification. Veins are generally closer to the surface than arteries and the pressure in them is lower. Massage aids the circulation by assisting venous flow to the heart and the elimination of waste, thus lowering blood pressure and increasing the percentage of oxygen in the tissues.

Heart

The bright red oxygenated blood from the lungs is pumped through the pulmonary veins to the left atrium and ventricle of the heart, and from there via the aorta to the arteries and all parts of the body. Darker, deoxy-genated blood returns via the veins to the right atrium and ventricle of the heart, where it is pumped through the pulmonary arteries to the lungs for recycling.

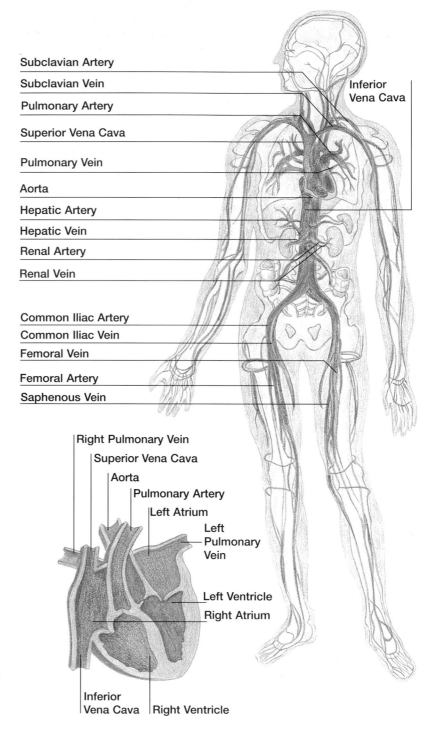

Subclavian Artery

Subclavian Vein

Pulmonary Artery

Superior Vena Cava

Pulmonary Vein

Aorta

Hepatic Artery

Hepatic Vein

Renal Artery

Renal Vein

Common Iliac Artery

Common Iliac Vein

Femoral Vein

Femoral Artery

Saphenous Vein

Inferior Vena Cava

Right Pulmonary Vein

Superior Vena Cava

Aorta

Pulmonary Artery

Left Atrium

Left Pulmonary Vein

Left Ventricle

Right Atrium

Inferior Vena Cava

Right Ventricle

Area drained
by Right
Lymphatic
Duct

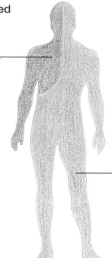

Lymph Drainage

Lymph comes originally from the blood.
When it has been cleared of impurities, it
is returned to the blood via two ducts: the
right lymphatic duct, which drains the
upper right-hand side of the body, and the
thoracic duct, which drains the remainder
of the body.

Area drained by
Thoracic Duct

Right Lymphatic Duct

Thoracic Duct

Lymph Vessel

Lymph Node

Lymphatic System

The lymphatic system helps to maintain the correct fluid balance in the tissues and blood, to defend the body against disease, to conserve protein and to remove bacteria and other cellular waste products. It is an intricate filtering system made up of tiny lymph vessels which circulate a milky fluid called lymph throughout the body. The movement of lymph is effected by the massage-like action of surrounding muscles, since the lymphatic system has no pump such as the heart to propel it. Lymph vessels carry excess fluid and bacteria from the tissues, which are then filtered out by lymph nodes or glands in the course of circulation. These nodes also produce the white blood cells known as lymphocytes. They are located along the vessels, rather like beads on a string. Clusters of nodes are found in the neck, armpits, groin and knees as well as down the middle of the torso, as shown right. Massage stimulates the lymphatic flow, and helps in the removal of lactic acid and other waste generated by excessive exercise.

The Nervous System

The nervous system receives inputs from internal and external stimuli, decodes and stores them in the brain, and generates behaviour in response. It consists of two parts – central and peripheral. The central nervous system comprises the brain and the spinal cord, and these form a two-way communication system linked with all other parts of the body via the peripheral nerves. The peripheral nervous system itself consists of two branches – voluntary (the spinal and cranial nerves) and the involuntary, or autonomic (responsible for functions such as digestion and respiration). There are two types of peripheral nerve cells, or neurons – sensory (or afferent) and motor (or efferent). The sensory neurons carry impulses from receptors in the sense organs to the spinal cord and brain; the motor neurons carry information and instructions from the brain to the organs and tissues via the spinal cord. Our nervous system allows us to appreciate and react appropriately to our environment; it also regulates the activities of the other bodily systems. By relaxing and toning the nerves, massage improves the condition of all the body's organs.

The Central and Peripheral Nervous Systems

The body's powerhouse is in the brain and spinal cord – the central nervous system. From the spine, the major nerves branch out to reach the body's periphery or extremities, forming the peripheral system. For the sake of clarity, the peripheral nerves have been greatly simplified in the illustration.

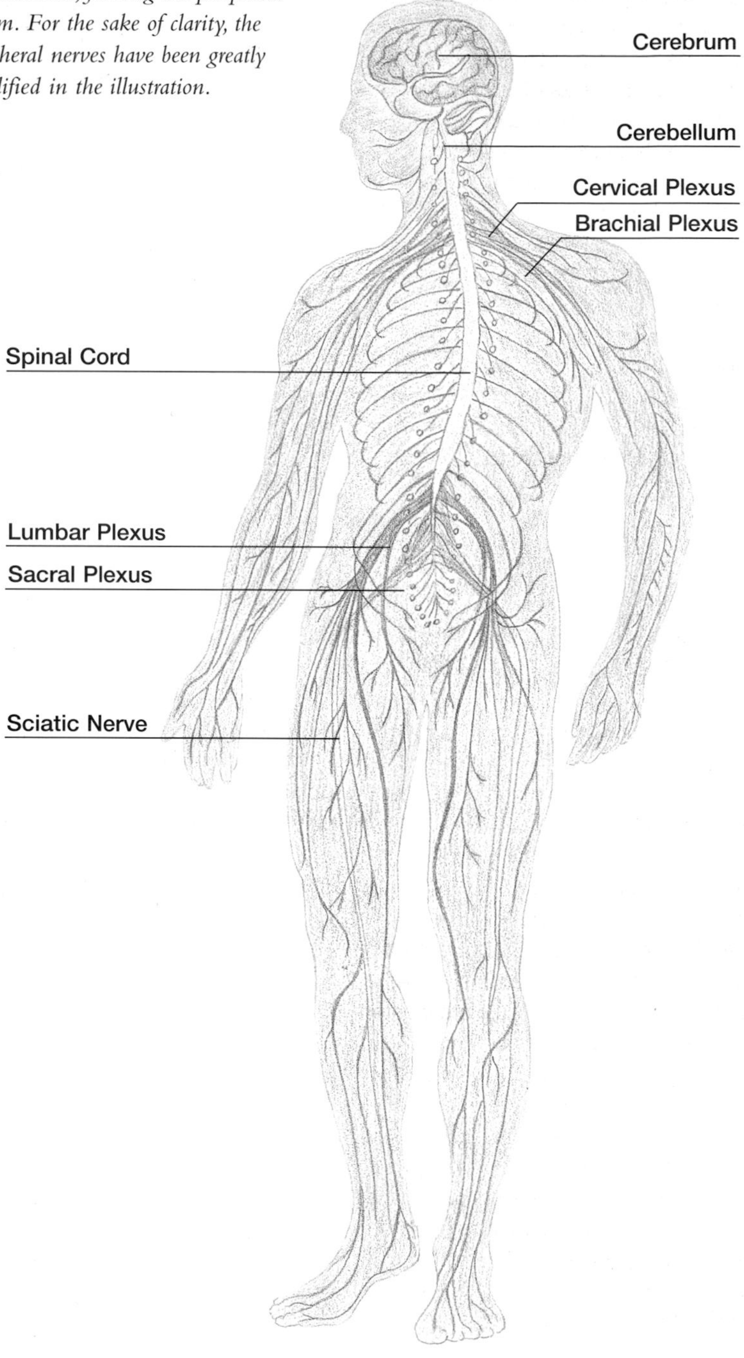

Cerebrum

Cerebellum

Cervical Plexus
Brachial Plexus

Spinal Cord

Lumbar Plexus

Sacral Plexus

Sciatic Nerve

Nerve Zones

The spinal nerves branch out from the spinal cord in pairs to service different parts of the body. The neck and arms are supplied by nerves from the cervical area; the ribcage and abdomen by nerves from the thoracic area; the lower back, hips and front of the legs by nerves from the lumbar area, and the backs of the legs by nerves from the sacral area. It is useful to understand which areas of the body are serviced by the various spinal nerves when giving massage, so that you can direct your treatment accordingly. If your partner has sciatic pain down one leg, for example, you should concentrate on the sacral area of the spine, as well as along the backs of the legs. Aching hip joints can be relieved at the lumbar area of the spine, as well as treated locally.

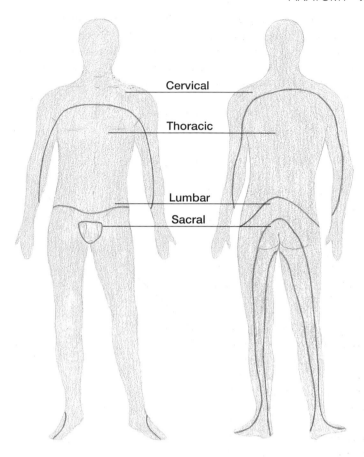

The Skin

The skin is the largest organ of the body – the organ of touch. It provides a strong protective waterproof covering for the underlying parts, and helps to eliminate waste and regulate temperature. Above all, it feeds us with information about the environment through its rich supply of nerve endings or receptor cells. Receptors that are sensitive to light touch, pain, heat and cold lie quite near the skin's surface, those activated by pressure are located farther in. The greatest number of receptors are those that are sensitive to pain, the smallest number are those sensitive to temperature. Also embedded in the skin are sweat glands which eliminate waste and help to cool the body through perspiration, and the sebaceous glands, which produce an oily secretion that lubricates the skin and protects it from bacteria.

The Structure of Skin

Skin consists of an outer layer of cells, the epidermis, and a thicker inner layer, the dermis. The epidermis, which is constantly being renewed, contains the receptor cells that respond to touch, while the dermis is supplied with the sebaceous and sweat glands. Under the dermis lies a layer of fat, known as subcutaneous tissue.

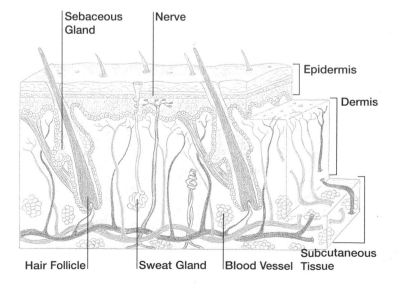

The Aura and Chakras

In addition to our physical anatomy, with its systems of circulation, respiration, and so on, there exists a "subtle" or psychic anatomy that is normally unseen. This subtle anatomy encompasses the aura that surrounds the physical body, and the major centres of psychic, or vital, energy known as chakras. The aura is generally described as an ovoid of luminous coloured emanations that interpenetrates and circulates around the physical body, as shown right. It is constantly in motion, reacting both to environmental inputs and to shifts in thought, feeling and physical well-being. The word "aura" literally means breeze and, indeed, to those that can see them, the shimmering layers of energy of which the aura is constituted do appear to move as if blown by the wind. Within the aura lie seven main chakras (shown opposite), which serve to relay the vital energy.

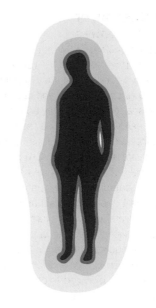

The Aura

The field of energy known as the aura is composed of three layers: the etheric, the astral, and the spiritual or causal bodies. The etheric body emanates out about 2–3 centimetres (1 inch) from the physical body. Its basic function is to receive and transmit vital energy – the life force known as *prana* in Sanskrit, *ki* in Japanese. The astral body extends a third of a metre (a foot) or more out around the body. It relates to the individual's emotional state and thought patterns, and it is through this body that we sense the moods or "vibrations" of other people. Negative thinking or unresolved emotions can filter down from this part of the aura to the etheric and physical levels, becoming manifest as disease. Extending out still farther from the body is the finest part of the aura, known as the spiritual or causal body. This may extend from a metre (a few feet) to hundreds of metres (hundreds of yards), depending on the spiritual evolution of the individual.

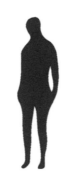 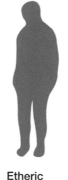 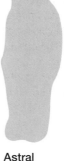 

Physical   **Etheric**   **Astral**   **Spiritual or Causal**

The Auric Bodies

The individual is made up of a physical body and an aura of subtle bodies – etheric, astral, and spiritual or causal. The physical body consists of matter of the densest and slowest vibrations, the spiritual body of subtle energy of the finest and fastest vibrations. All four bodies interpenetrate with one another to form a subtle energy field, as shown above.

Chakra Sanskrit name	**Root** *Muladhara*
Gland	Adrenals
Physical parts and organs governed	Legs; feet; genitals; anus; coccyx; kidneys
Realm of behaviour and human development	Physical will to be; primordial origins; survival

The Chakras or Energy Centres

The seven chakras are centres of energy in the etheric body. To sensitives who can see them, they appear as whirling, cone-shaped vortices or as saucer-shaped depressions, according to the health and spiritual development of the individual. But even those of us who cannot see them can learn to sense their individual energies with our hands. Located along the spine, as shown right, the chakras act as the main receivers and distributors of vital energy between the physical body and the subtle bodies of the aura. Each chakra corresponds to a different gland and governs specific parts of the physical body and areas of psychological and spiritual development, as shown on the chart below. Balance between the chakras results in maximum vitality and health. Damage to one of the chakras or subtle bodies through physical or emotional trauma will be manifested as dysfunction in the relative areas of the body. The aim of healing arts such as acupuncture, shiatsu, and massage is to restore the individual's balance of energies and to bring him or her into harmony with the universal pulse of life.

The Seven Chakras

The chakras can be perceived both at the back and the front of the body – from the Root Chakra at the base of the spine to the Crown Chakra at the top of the head. They are often conceived of as lotuses, each with a different number of petals representing the energy channels that flow through them. The Crown Chakra is said to have one thousand petals.

Hara	**Solar Plexus**	**Heart**	**Throat**	**Brow**	**Crown**
Swadhisthana	*Manipura*	*Anahata*	*Vishuddha*	*Ajna*	*Sahasrara*
Gonads	Pancreas	Thymus	Thyroid	Pituitary	Pineal
Pelvis; genitals; reproductive system; belly; sacrum; lumbar vertebrae	Lumbar vertebrae; stomach; gall bladder; liver; diaphragm; nervous system	Heart; lower lungs; chest; breasts; thoracic vertebrae; circulatory system	Arms; hands; throat; mouth; voice; lungs; cervical vertebrae; respiratory system	Forehead; ears; nose; left eye; base of skull; medulla; nervous system	Cranium; cerebral cortex; right eye
Vitality; movement; sexual expression; grounding	Raw emotional energy; desire; personal power	Love; compassion; service to humanity	Self-expression; creativity; clairaudience	Intuition; intellect; clairvoyance	Transcendence; superconsciousness; spiritual will to be

Recommended Reading

For massage and touch:
Downing, George, *The Massage Book*, Penguin, 1972
Juhan, Deane, *Job's Body*, Station Hill Press, 1987
Knaster, Mirka, *Discovering the Body's Wisdom*,
    Bantam Books, 1996
Maxwell-Hudson, Clare, *The Complete Illustrated
    Guide to Massage*, Dorling Kindersley, 1999
Montagu, Ashley, *Touching*, Harper & Row, 1971
Thomas, Sara, *Massage for Common Ailments*, Gaia
    Books, 1989

For shiatsu:
Beresford-Cooke, Carola, *Shiatsu Theory and Practice*,
    Churchill Livingstone, 1996
Liechti, Elaine, *The Complete Illustrated Guide to
    Shiatsu*, Element Books, 1998
Lundberg, Paul, *The Book of Shiatsu*, Gaia Books,
    1992
Masunaga, Shizuto, *Zen Shiatsu*, Japan Publications,
    1977

For reflexology:
Byers, Dwight C., *Better Health with Foot Reflexology*,
    Ingham Publishing, 1983
Ingham, Eunice D., *Stories the Feet Can Tell*, Ingham
    Publishing, 1938; *Stories the Feet Have Told*, Ingham
    Publishing, 1951

For baby massage:
Leboyer, Frederick, *Loving Hands*, Newmarket Press,
    1976
Walker, Peter, *Baby Massage*, Piatkus, 1995

For body reading:
Dychtwald, Ken, *Bodymind*, Tarcher Putnam, 1995.

Useful Addresses

To obtain information about courses, workshops or
individual treatments, please contact one of the following:

For massage: UK
Sara Thomas
15A Bridge Avenue
London W6 9JA

Lucy Lidell
c/o Gaia Books
20 High Street
Stroud
Gloucestershire GL5 1AS

The Massage Training Institute
    (MTI)
90–92 Islington High Street
London N1 8EG

Massage Therapy Institute GB
PO Box 276
London NW2 4NR

**For massage tables and
accessories: UK**
New Concept
2 Bermuda Road
Ransome's Euro Park
Ipswich, Suffolk IP3 9RU

Oakworks
Avon Road
Charfield, Wotton-under-Edge
Gloucestershire GL12 8TT

The Tavy Cover
Kimberleigh
Bolt House Close
Tavistock, Devon PL19 8LN

For massage: USA
Esalen Massage and Bodywork
    Association
Highway 1
Big Sur, CA 93920

Boulder College of Massage
    Therapy
6255 Longbow Drive
Boulder, CO 80301

See also *Resource Guide*
Noah Publishing
PO Box 1500
Davis, CA 95617-1500

**For massage tables and
accessories: USA**
See *Massage Magazine*
13115 West Mallon Avenue
Spokane, WA 99201

**For massage research:
USA**
Touch Research Institute
University of Miami
PO Box 016720
Miami, FL 33101

For shiatsu: UK
Carola Beresford-Cooke
c/o Health Matters
4 Chancery Lane
Cardigan SA43 1HD

The Shiatsu Society
Eastlands Court
St Peter's Road
Rugby CV21 3QP

For shiatsu: USA
American Oriental Bodywork
    Therapy Association
50 Maple Place, Manhasset
New York, NY 11030

Pauline Sasaki
260 West Cedar Street
Norwalk
Connecticut, CT 06854/1330

For reflexology: UK
International Institute of
    Reflexology
255 Turleigh, Bradford-on-Avon
Wiltshire BA15 2HG

Advanced Reflexology Training
    (ART)
28 Hollyfield Avenue
London N11 3BY

For reflexology: USA
International Institute of
    Reflexology
PO Box 12642
St Petersburg
Florida, FL 33733-2642

Index

A

Abdomen 71, 122–5
Ampuku 122–5
Anatomy 180–9
Ankle Rotation Technique 139
Appendix Reflex 144
Arms 63–7, 118–21
Ascending Colon Reflex 144
Aura 188

B

Babies 156–9
Back 40–5, 92–5
Back and Forth Technique 139
Bladder Meridian 92, 95, 96, 98, 100,
    106, 110, 112, 114
Body Reading 166–79
Bones 180
Broad Circling 31
Brow Chakra 189
Buttocks 44, 172

C

Centring 24–5
Chakras 189
Chest 70, 111, 174
    see also Torso
Circulation 184
Connecting 76–7
Contraindications 36, 90, 138
Crown Chakra 189
Cupping 35

D

Deep Tissue Strokes 33
Descending Colon Reflex 144
Diaphragm and Solar Plexus Flexing
    Technique 139
Diaphragm Line 135, 136–7
"Dragon's Mouth" Hold 89

E

Ear Reflex 142
Earth Element 83, 126
Eye Reflex 142

F

Face 58–62, 114–17, 177

Feathering 31
Feet 50–1, 75, 104–5, 134–47, 170
Fire Element 83, 118
Five Elements 83
Foot Reflexes Chart 136–7
Foot Treatment Sequence 142–7

G

Gall Bladder Meridian 96, 100, 106
Giving and Receiving 22
Gliding Strokes 30–1
Governing Vessel 85, 110, 112, 114
"Great Eliminator" 121, 155
Grounding 170

H

Hacking 35
Hand Reflexology 148–51
Hands 63–7, 118–21
Hara 24, 88, 122–5, 172–3, 189
Head 114–17
Head Reflex 142
Heart 184
Heart Chakra 189
Heart Meridian 118
Heart Protector 118
Heel Line 135
Hip/Knee/Leg Reflex 147, 151
Hip Reflex 147
Hips 44, 96–9
History 10, 12
Holding Techique 140
Hooking 141

I

Ileocecal Valve Reflex 144
Index Finger Technique 141
Ingham, Eunice 132

J

Jitsu 81, 85, 110
Joints 180

K

Ki 81, 82–5, 86
Kidney Meridian 100, 111
Kneading 32
Kyo 81, 85, 110

L

Legs 171
    Back of 46–9, 100–105
    Front of 72–5, 126–9
Liver Meridian 126
Liver Reflex 144, 151
Long Stroke 30
Lung Meridian 110, 111, 118
Lung Reflex 143, 150
Lymphatic System 185

M

Massage 16, 27–79
    basic sequence 36–7
    basic strokes 30–5
    checklist 78–9
    Swedish 12, 27
Masunaga, Shizuto 81, 114
Meridians 81, 85, 92, 96, 100, 106,
    110, 114, 121, 122, 126
    see also individual meridians
Metal Element 83, 118
"Mother" Hand 102
Muscles 182–3

N

Neck 43, 54, 112–13, 176
Neck Reflex 143
Nervous System 186–7

O

Oiling 28–9
Oils 28

P

Padding 38–9
Pelvis 172
Percussion 35
Plucking 35
Pressure Points (for Massage) 131
    see also Tsubos
Pulling 32
Pummelling 35

R

Referral Areas 163
Reflexology 16, 132–51
    basic techniques 138–41

Index (continued)

Reflex Rotation 141
Root Chakra 172, 189

S
Sacrum 98
Shiatsu 16, 80–131
  basic sequence 90–1
  basic techniques 88–9
  checklist 130
Shoulders 42–3, 52–7, 65, 66, 175
  Back of 106–9
  Front of 110–13
Sigmoid Colon Reflex 144
Sinus Reflex 142
Skeleton 180–1
Skin 187
Small Intestine Meridian 106, 108,
  110, 114, 118
Solar Plexus Chakra 189
Spinal Reflexes 146, 151
Spine 42, 45, 56
Spleen Meridian 110, 126
Stomach Meridian 110, 111, 114, 126
Stomach 36 126, 128, 155

T
Tan-Den 24, 122, 124
Throat Chakra 189
Thumb Pressure 89
Thumb-rolling 33
Thumb Technique 140
Torso, Front of 68–71
Towels 38–9
Triple Heater 110, 114, 118
Tsubos 81, 85, 89, 131

W
Waist Line 135, 136–7, 148–9
Water Element 83, 100
Wood Element 83, 100
Working Surfaces 20
Wringing 32

Y
Yin and Yang 82, 83, 85

Z
Zone Theory 134

Acknowledgments

Gaia would like to extend thanks to the following:

Hylton Allcock; Miranda Allcock; Janey Arnold; Sharon Bannister; Irma Basson; Carola Beresford-Cooke; Terry Bryan; Peter Camp; Jeoff Canin; Nicky Childs; Elizabeth Courtier; Peter Courtier; Guy Dartnell; Hélène Debargé; Fausto Dorelli; Billy Doyle; Geraldine; Duncan Gillies; Jerry Gloag; Usha Gundelach; David Hamilton; Liz Hood; Jeremy Hopkins; Joni; Len Joseph; Michael Lewis; Jan Liberadski; Lucy Lidell; Elaine Liechti; Miren Lopategui; Agnes Maurer; Clare Maxwell-Hudson; Penny Allen; William McEwan; Anne Neary; Anthony Porter; Katy Pring; Roger Pring; Sally Pring; Sarah Pring; Phil Reynolds; Corinne Roché; Michael Rose; Kali Rosenblum; Michael Selby; Kevin Smith; Peter Sperryn; Nigel Stainton; Tom Sturgess-Lief; Sara Thomas; Ann Vadgama; Laural Wade; Claire Warburton; Sarah Webster; Rosie Wildwood

and special thanks to Ann Parks for the inspiration of her teaching.

Illustrators
Sheila Hadley; Sylvia Kwan; Sheilagh Noble; Joe Robinson

Picture credits
Egyptian wall-painting (p. 13): International Institute of Reflexology; Illustration from Avicenna's *Canon* (p. 13); Joseph Regenstein Library, University of Chicago, Illinois; Illustration from *Ampuku zukai*: Ido No Nipponsha, Tokyo (p. 13).

Typesetting
Aardvark Editorial Ltd
Mendham, Suffolk

Colour origination
L.C. Repro Ltd, Aldermaston